BODY RESET DIET

THE FULL BODY RESET

Return Your Body to
Peak Metabolism

LAILAH TURNER

Table of Contents

PART I

Reset Diet

In this chapter, we are going to study the details of the reset diet and what recipes you can make.

Chapter 1: How to Reset Your Body?

Created by a celebrity trainer, Harley Pasternak, the body reset diet is a famous fifteen-day eating pattern that aims to jump-start weight loss. According to Pasternak, if you experience rapid loss in weight early in a diet, you will feel more motivated to stick to that diet plan. This theory is even supported by a few scientific studies (Alice A Gibson, 2017).

The body reset diet claims to help in weight loss with light exercise and low-calorie diet plans for fifteen days. The diet is divided into 3 phases of five days each. Each phase had a particular pattern of diet and exercise routine. You need to consume food five times every day, starting from the first phase, which mostly consists of smoothies and progressing to more solid foods in the second and third phases.

The three phases of the body reset diet are:

- **Phase One** – During this stage, you are required to consume only two snacks every day and drink smoothies for breakfast, lunch, and dinner. In the case of exercise, you have to walk at least ten thousand steps per day.

- **Phase Two** – During this phase, you can eat two snacks each day, consume solid food only once, and have to replace any two meals of the day with smoothies. In case of exercise, apart from walking ten thousand steps every day, on three of the days, you also have to finish five minutes of resistance training with the help of four separate exercises.

- **Phase Three** – You can consume two snacks every day, but you have to eat two low-calorie meals and replace one of your meals with a smoothie. For exercise, you are required to walk ten thousand steps. Apart from that, you also have to finish five minutes of resistance training with the help of four separate exercises each day.

After you have finished the standard fifteen-day diet requirements, you have to keep following the meal plan you followed in the third phase. However, during this time, you are allowed to have two "free meals" twice a week in which you can consume anything you want. These "free meals" are meant as a reward so that you can avoid feeling deprived. According to Pasternak, depriving yourself of a particular food continuously can result in binge eating (Nawal Alajmi, 2016).

There is no official endpoint of the diet after the first fifteen days for losing and maintaining weight. Pasternak suggests that the habits and routines formed over fifteen days should be maintained for a lifetime.

Chapter 2: Science Behind Metabolism Reset

Several people take on a "cleanse" or "detox" diet every year to lose the extra holiday weight or simply start following healthy habits. However, some fat diet plans are often a bit overwhelming. For example, it requires a tremendous amount of self-discipline to drink only juices. Moreover, even after finishing a grueling detox diet plan, you might just go back to eating foods that are bad for you because of those days of deprivation. New studies issued in the *Medicine & Science in Sports & Exercise* shows that low-calorie diets may result in binge eating, which is not the right method for lasting weight loss.

Another research conducted by the researchers at Loughborough University showed that healthy, college-aged women who followed a calorie-restricted diet consumed an extra three hundred calories at dinner as compared to the control group who consumed three standard meals. They revealed that it was because they had lower levels of peptide YY (represses appetite) and higher levels of ghrelin (makes you hungry). They are most likely to go hog wild when you are feeling ravenous, and it's finally time to eat (Nawal Alajmi K. D.-O., 2016).

Another research published in *Cognitive Neuroscience* studied the brains of chronic dieters. They revealed that there was a weaker connection between the two regions of the brain in people who had a higher percentage of body fat. They showed that they might have an increased risk of getting obese because it's harder for them to set their temptations aside (Pin-Hao Andy Chen, 2016).

A few other studies, however, also revealed that you could increase your self-control through practice. Self-control, similar to any other kind of strength, also requires time to develop. However, you can consider focusing on a diet plan that can help you "reset" instead of putting all your efforts into developing your self-control to get healthy.

A reset is considered as a new start – one that can get your metabolism and your liver in good shape. The liver is the biggest solid organ of your body, and it's mainly responsible for removing toxins that can harm your health and well-being by polluting your system. Toxins keep accumulating in your body all the time, and even though it's the liver's job to handle this, it can sometimes get behind schedule, which can result in inflammation. It causes a lot of strain on your metabolism and results in weight gain, particularly around the abdomen. The best method to alleviate this inflammation is to follow a metabolism rest diet and give your digestive system a vacation (Olivia M. Farr, 2015).

Chapter 3: Recipes for Smoothies and Salads

If you want to lose weight and you have a particular period within which you want to achieve it, then here are some recipes that are going to be helpful.

Green Smoothie

Total Prep & Cooking Time: 2 minutes

Yields: 1 serving

Nutrition Facts: Calories: 144 | Carbs: 28.2g | Protein: 3.4g | Fat: 2.9g | Fiber: 4.8g

Ingredients:

- One cup each of
  - Almond milk
  - Raw spinach
- One-third of a cup of strawberries
- One orange, peeled

Method:

1. Add the peeled orange, strawberries, almond milk, and raw spinach in a blender and blend everything until you get a smooth paste. You can add extra water if required to achieve the desired thickness.

2. Pour out the smoothie into a glass and serve.

Strawberry Banana Smoothie

Total Prep & Cooking Time: 5 minutes

Yields: 2 servings

Nutrition Facts: Calories: 198| Carbs: 30.8g | Protein: 5.9g | Fat: 7.1g | Fiber: 4.8g

Ingredients:

- Half a cup each of
  - Milk
  - Greek yogurt
- One banana, frozen and quartered
- Two cups of fresh strawberries, halved

Method:

1. Add the milk, Greek yogurt, banana, and strawberries into a high-powered blender and blend until you get a smooth mixture.

2. Pour the smoothie equally into two separate glasses and serve.

Notes:

- *Don't add ice to the smoothie as it can make it watery very quickly. Using frozen bananas will keep your smoothie cold.*

- *As you're using bananas and strawberries, there is no need to add any artificial sweetener.*

Salmon Citrus Salad

Total Prep & Cooking Time: 20 minutes

Yields: 6 servings

Nutrition Facts: Calories: 336 | Carbs: 20g | Protein: 17g | Fat: 21g | Fiber: 5g

Ingredients:

- One pound of Citrus Salmon (slow-roasted)
- Half of an English cucumber, sliced
- One tomato (large), sliced into a quarter of an inch thick pieces
- One grapefruit, peeled and cut into segments
- Two oranges, peeled and cut into segments
- Three beets, roasted and quartered
- One avocado
- Boston lettuce leaves
- Two tablespoons of red wine vinegar
- Half of a red onion
- Flakey salt
- Aleppo pepper flakes

For the Citrus Shallot Vinaigrette,

- Five tablespoons of olive oil (extra-virgin)
- One clove of garlic, smashed
- Salt and pepper
- One and a half tablespoons of rice wine vinegar
- Two tablespoons of orange juice or fresh lemon juice
- One tablespoon of shallot, minced

Method:

For preparing the Citrus Shallot Vinaigrette:

1. Add the ingredients for the vinaigrette in a bowl and whisk them together.

2. Keep the mixture aside.

For assembling the salad,

1. Add the onions and vinegar in a small bowl and pickle them by letting them sit for about fifteen minutes.

2. In the meantime, place the lettuce leaves on the serving plate.

3. Dice the avocado in half and eliminate the pit. Then scoop the flesh and add them onto the plate. Sprinkle a dash of flakey salt and Aleppo pepper on top to season it.

4. Add the quartered beets onto the serving plate along with the grapefruit and orange segments.

5. Salt the cucumber and tomato slices lightly and add them onto the plate.

6. Then, scatter the pickled onions on top and cut the salmon into bits and add it on the plate.

7. Lastly, drizzle the Citrus Shallot Vinaigrette on top of the salad and finish off with a dash of flakey salt.

Chapter 4: Quick and Easy Breakfast and Main Course Recipes

Quinoa Salad
Total Prep & Cooking Time: 40 minutes

Yields: Eight servings

Nutrition Facts: Calories: 205 | Carbs: 25.9g | Protein: 6.1g | Fat: 9.4g | Fiber: 4.6g

Ingredients:

- One tablespoon of red wine vinegar
- One-fourth of a cup each of
    - Lemon juice (about two to three lemons)
    - Olive oil
- One cup each of
    - Quinoa (uncooked), rinsed with the help of a fine-mesh colander
    - Flat-leaf parsley (from a single large bunch), finely chopped
- Three-fourth of a cup of red onion (one small red onion), chopped
- One red bell pepper (medium-sized), chopped
- One cucumber (medium-sized), seeded and chopped
- One and a half cups of chickpeas (cooked), or One can of chickpeas (about fifteen ounces), rinsed and drained
- Two cloves of garlic, minced or pressed
- Two cups of water
- Black pepper, freshly ground
- Half a teaspoon of fine sea salt

Method:

1. Place a medium-sized saucepan over medium-high heat and add the rinsed quinoa into it along with the water. Allow the mixture to boil and then reduce the heat and simmer it. Cook for about fifteen minutes so that the quinoa has absorbed all the water. As time goes on, decrease the heat and maintain a gentle simmer. Take the saucepan away from the heat and cover it with a lid. Allow the cooked quinoa to rest for about five minutes to give it some time to increase in size.

2. Add the onions, bell pepper, cucumber, chickpeas, and parsley in a large serving bowl and mix them together. Keep the mixture aside.

3. Add the garlic, vinegar, lemon juice, olive oil, and salt in another small bowl and whisk the ingredients so that they are appropriately combined. Keep this mixture aside.

4. When the cooked quinoa has almost cooled down, transfer it to the serving bowl. Add the dressing on top and toss to combine everything together.

5. Add an extra pinch of sea salt and the black pepper to season according to your preference. Allow the salad to rest for five to ten minutes before serving it for the best results.

6. You can keep the salad in the refrigerator for up to four days. Make sure to cover it properly.

7. You can serve it at room temperature or chilled.

Notes: Instead of cooking additional quinoa, you can use about three cups of leftover quinoa for making this salad. Moreover, you can also serve this salad with fresh greens and an additional drizzle of lemon juice and olive oil. You can also add a dollop of cashew sour cream or crumbled feta cheese as a topping.

Herb and Goat Cheese Omelet

Total Prep & Cooking Time: 20 minutes

Yields: Two servings

Nutrition Facts: Calories: 233 | Carbs: 3.6g | Protein: 16g | Fat: 17.6g | Fiber: 1g

Ingredients:

- Half a cup each of
  - Red bell peppers (3 x quarter-inch), julienne-cut
  - Zucchini, thinly sliced
- Four large eggs
- Two teaspoons of olive oil, divided
- One-fourth of a cup of goat cheese (one ounce), crumbled
- Half a teaspoon of fresh tarragon, chopped
- One teaspoon each of
  - Fresh parsley, chopped
  - Fresh chives, chopped
- One-eighth of a teaspoon of salt
- One-fourth of a teaspoon of black pepper, freshly ground (divided)
- One tablespoon of water

Method:

1. Break the eggs into a bowl and add one tablespoon of water into it. Whisk them together and add in one-eighth of a teaspoon each of salt and ground black pepper.

2. In another small bowl, mix the goat cheese, tarragon, and parsley and keep it aside.

3. Place a nonstick skillet over medium heat and heat one teaspoon of olive oil in it. Add in the sliced zucchini, bell pepper, and the remaining one-eighth of a teaspoon of black pepper along with a dash of salt. Cook for about four minutes so that the bell pepper and zucchini get soft. Transfer the zucchini-bell pepper mixture onto a plate and cover it with a lid to keep it warm.

4. Add about half a teaspoon of oil into a skillet and add in half of the whisked egg into it. Do not stir the eggs and let the egg set slightly. Loosen the set edges of the omelet carefully with the help of a spatula. Tilt the skillet to move the uncooked part of the egg to the side. Keep following this method for about five seconds so that there is no more runny egg in the skillet. Add half of the crumbled goat cheese mixture evenly over the omelet and let it cook for another minute so that it sets.

5. Transfer the omelet onto a plate and fold it into thirds.

6. Repeat the process with the rest of the egg mixture, half a teaspoon of olive oil, and the goat cheese mixture.

7. Add the chopped chives on top of the omelets and serve with the bell pepper and zucchini mixture.

Mediterranean Cod

Total Prep & Cooking Time: 15 minutes

Yields: 4 servings

Nutrition Facts: Calories: 320 | Carbs: 31g | Protein: 35g | Fat: 8g | Fiber: 8g

Ingredients:

- One pound of spinach
- Four fillets of cod (almost one and a half pounds)
- Two zucchinis (medium-sized), chopped
- One cup of marinara sauce
- One-fourth of a teaspoon of red pepper, crushed
- Two cloves of garlic, chopped
- One tablespoon of olive oil
- Salt and pepper, according to taste
- Whole wheat roll, for serving

Method:

1. Place a ten-inch skillet on medium heat and add the marinara sauce and zucchini into it. Combine them together and let it simmer on medium heat.

2. Add the fillets of cod into the simmering sauce. Add one-fourth of a teaspoon each of salt and pepper too. Cover the skillet with a lid and let it cook for about seven minutes so that the cod gets just opaque throughout.

3. In the meantime, place a five-quart saucepot on medium heat and heat the olive oil in it. Add in the crushed red pepper and minced garlic. Stir and cook for about a minute.

4. Then, add in the spinach along with one-eighth of a teaspoon of salt. Cover the saucepot with a lid and let it cook for about five minutes, occasionally stirring so that the spinach gets wilted.

5. Add the spinach on the plates and top with the sauce and cod mixture and serve with the whole wheat roll.

Grilled Chicken and Veggies

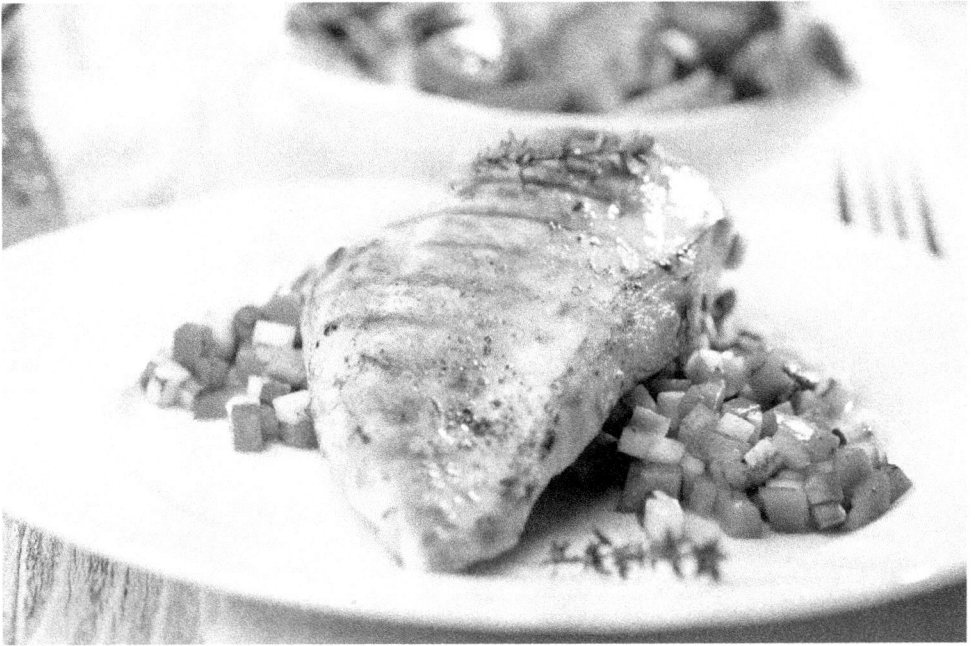

Total Prep & Cooking Time: 35 minutes

Yields: 4 servings

Nutrition Facts: Calories: 305 | Carbs: 11g | Protein: 26g | Fat: 17g | Fiber: 3g

Ingredients:

For the marinade,

- Four cloves of garlic, crushed

- One-fourth of a cup each of
  - Fresh lemon juice
  - Olive oil
- One teaspoon each of
  - Salt
  - Smoked paprika
  - Dried oregano
- Black pepper, according to taste
- Half a teaspoon of red chili flakes

For the grilling,

- Two to three zucchinis or courgette (large), cut into thin slices
- Twelve to sixteen spears of asparagus, woody sides trimmed
- Broccoli
- Two bell peppers, seeds eliminated and cut into thin slices
- Four pieces of chicken breasts (large), skinless and de-boned

Method:

1. Preheat your griddle or grill pan.

2. Sprinkle some salt on top of the chicken breasts to season them. Keep them aside to rest while you prepare the marinade.

3. For the marinade, mix all the ingredients properly.

4. Add about half of the marinade over the vegetables and the other half over the seasoned chicken breasts. Allow the marinade to rest for a couple of minutes.

5. Place the chicken pieces on the preheated grill. Grill for about five to seven minutes on each side until they are cooked according to your preference. The time on the grill depends on the thickness of the chicken breasts.

6. Remove them from the grill and cover them using a foil. Set it aside to rest and prepare to grill the vegetables in the meantime.

7. Grill the vegetables for a few minutes until they begin to char and are crispy yet tender.

8. Remove them from the grill and transfer them onto a serving plate. Serve the veggies along with the grilled chicken and add the lemon wedges on the side for squeezing.

Notes: *You can add as much or as little vegetables as you like. The vegetable amounts are given only as a guide. Moreover, feel free to replace some of them with the vegetables you like to eat.*

Stuffed Peppers

Total Prep & Cooking Time: 50 minutes

Yields: 4 servings

Nutrition Facts: Calories: 438 | Carbs: 32g | Protein: 32g | Fat: 20g | Fiber: 5g

Ingredients:

For the stuffed peppers,

- One pound of ground chicken or turkey
- Four bell peppers (large) of any color
- One and a quarter of a cups of cheese, shredded
- One and a half cups of brown rice, cooked (you can use cauliflower rice or quinoa)
- One can (about fourteen ounces) of fire-roasted diced tomatoes along with its juices
- Two teaspoons of olive oil (extra-virgin)
- One teaspoon each of
  o Garlic powder
  o Ground cumin
- One tablespoon of ground chili powder
- One-fourth of a teaspoon of black pepper
- Half a teaspoon of kosher salt

For serving,

- Sour cream or Greek yogurt

- Salsa

- Freshly chopped cilantro

- Avocado, sliced

- Freshly squeezed lemon juice

Method:

1. Preheat your oven to 375 degrees Fahrenheit.

2. Take a nine by thirteen-inch baking dish and coat it lightly with a nonstick cooking spray.

3. Take the bell peppers and slice them from top to bottom into halves. Remove the membranes and the seeds. Keep the bell peppers in the baking dish with the cut-side facing upwards.

4. Place a large, nonstick skillet on medium-high heat and heat the olive oil in it. Add in the chicken, pepper, salt, garlic powder, ground cumin, and chili powder and cook for about four minutes so that the chicken is cooked through and gets brown. Break apart the chicken while it's cooking. Drain off any excess liquid and then add in the can of diced tomatoes along with the juices. Allow it to simmer for a minute.

5. Take the pan away from the heat. Add in the cooked rice along with three-fourth of a cup of the shredded cheese and stir everything together.

6. Add this filling inside the peppers and add the remaining shredded cheese as a topping.

7. Add a little amount of water into the pan containing the peppers so that it barely covers the bottom of the pan.

8. Keep it uncovered and bake it in the oven for twenty-five to thirty-five minutes so that the cheese gets melted and the peppers get soft.

9. Add any of your favorite fixings as a topping and serve hot.

Notes:

- *For preparing the stuffed peppers ahead of time, make sure to allow the rice and chicken mixture to cool down completely before filling the peppers. You can prepare the stuffed peppers before time, and then you have to cover it with a lid and keep it in the refrigerator for a maximum of twenty-four hours before baking the peppers.*

- *If you're planning to reheat the stuffed peppers, gently reheat them in your oven or microwave. If you're using a microwave for this purpose, make sure to cut the peppers into pieces to warm them evenly.*

- *You can store any leftovers in the freezer for up to three months. Alternatively, you can keep them in the refrigerator for up to four days. Allow it to thaw in the fridge overnight.*

Brussels Sprouts With Honey Mustard Chicken

Total Prep & Cooking Time: Fifty minutes

Yields: Four servings

Nutrition Facts: Calories: 360 | Carbs: 14.5g | Protein: 30.8g | Fat: 20g | Fiber: 3.7g

Ingredients:

- One and a half pounds of Brussels sprouts, divided into two halves
- Two pounds of chicken thighs, skin-on and bone-in (about four medium-sized thighs)
- Three cloves of garlic, minced
- One-fourth of a large onion, cut into slices
- One tablespoon each of
  - Honey
  - Whole-grain mustard
  - Dijon mustard
- Two tablespoons of freshly squeezed lemon juice (one lemon)
- One-fourth of a cup plus two tablespoons of olive oil (extra-virgin)
- Freshly ground black pepper
- Kosher salt
- Non-stick cooking spray

Method:

1. Preheat your oven to 425 degrees Fahrenheit.

2. Take a large baking sheet and grease it with nonstick cooking spray. Keep it aside.

3. Add the minced garlic, honey, whole-grain mustard, Dijon mustard, one tablespoon of the lemon juice, one-fourth cup of the olive oil in a medium-sized bowl and mix them together. Add the Kosher salt and black pepper to season according to your preference.

4. Dip the chicken thighs into the sauce with the help of tongs and coat both sides. Transfer the things on the baking sheet. You can get rid of any extra sauce.

5. Mix the red onion and Brussels sprouts in a medium-sized bowl and drizzle one tablespoon of lemon juice along with the remaining two tablespoons of olive oil onto it. Toss everything together until the vegetables are adequately coated.

6. Place the red onion-Brussels sprouts mixture on the baking sheet around the chicken pieces. Ensure that the chicken and vegetables are not overlapping.

7. Sprinkle a little amount of salt and pepper on the top and keep it in the oven to roast for about thirty to thirty-five minutes so that the Brussels sprouts get crispy and the chicken has an internal temperature of 165 degrees Fahrenheit and has turned golden brown.

8. Serve hot.

Quinoa Stuffed Chicken

Total Prep & Cooking Time: 50 minutes

Yields: Four servings

Nutrition Facts: Calories: 355 | Carbs: 28g | Protein: 30g | Fat: 13g | Fiber: 4g

Ingredients:

- One and a half cups of chicken broth
- Three-fourths of a cup of quinoa (any color of your choice)
- Four chicken breasts (boneless and skinless)
- One lime, zested and one tablespoon of lime juice
- One-fourth of a cup of cilantro, chipped
- One-third of a cup of unsweetened coconut, shaved or coconut chips
- One Serrano pepper, seeded and diced
- Two cloves of garlic, minced
- Half a cup of red onion, diced
- Three-fourth of a cup of bell pepper, diced
- One tablespoon of coconut oil
- One teaspoon each of
  - Salt
  - Chili powder
  - Ground cumin

Method:

1. Preheat your oven to 375 degrees Fahrenheit.

2. Take a rimmed baking sheet and line it with parchment paper.

3. Place a medium-sized saucepan over medium-high heat and add the coconut oil in it. After it has melted, add in the Serrano peppers, garlic, red onion, and bell pepper and sauté for about one to two minutes so that they soften just a bit. Make sure that the vegetables are still bright in color. Then transfer the cooked vegetables into a bowl.

4. Add the quinoa in the empty sauce pot and increase the heat to high. Pour the chicken broth in it along with half a teaspoon of salt. Close the lid of the pot and bring it to a boil, allowing the quinoa to cook for about fifteen minutes so that the surface of the quinoa develops vent holes, and the broth has absorbed completely. Take the pot away from the heat and allow it to steam for an additional five minutes.

5. In the meantime, cut a slit along the long side in each chicken breast. It will be easier with the help of a boning knife. You are making a deep pocket in each breast, having a half-inch border around the remaining three attached sides. Keep the knife parallel to the cutting board and cut through the middle of the breast and leaving the opposite side attached. Try to cut it evenly as it's challenging to cook thick uncut portions properly in the oven. After that, add salt, cumin, and chili powder on all sides of the chicken.

6. When the quinoa has turned fluffy, add in the lime juice, lime zest, shaved coconut, and sautéed vegetables and stir them in. Taste the mixture and adjust the salt as per your preference.

7. Add the confetti quinoa mixture inside the cavity of the chicken breast. Place the stuffed breasts on the baking sheet with the quinoa facing upwards. They'll look like open envelopes.

8. Bake them in the oven for about twenty minutes.

9. Serve warm.

Kale and Sweet Potato Frittata

Total Prep & Cooking Time: 30 minutes

Yields: 4 servings

Nutrition Facts: Calories: 144 | Carbs: 10g | Protein: 7g | Fat: 9g | Fiber: 2g

Ingredients:

- Three ounces of goat cheese
- Two cloves of garlic
- Half of a red onion (small)
- Two cups each of
  o Sweet potatoes
  o Firmly packed kale, chopped
- Two tablespoons of olive oil
- One cup of half-and-half
- Six large eggs
- Half a teaspoon of pepper, freshly ground
- One teaspoon of Kosher salt

Method:

1. Preheat your oven to 350 degrees Fahrenheit.

2. Add the eggs, half-and-half, salt, and black pepper in a bowl and whisk everything together.

3. Place a ten-inch ovenproof nonstick skillet over medium heat and add one tablespoon of oil in it. Sauté the sweet potatoes in the skillet for about eight to ten minutes so that they turn soft and golden brown. Transfer them onto a plate and keep warm.

4. Next, add in the remaining one tablespoon of oil and sauté the kale along with the red onions and garlic in it for about three to four minutes so that the kale gets soft and wilted. Then, add in the whisked egg mixture evenly over the vegetables and cook for an additional three minutes.

5. Add some goat cheese on the top and bake it in the oven for ten to fourteen minutes so that it sets.

Walnut, Ginger, and Pineapple Oatmeal

Total Prep & Cooking Time: 30 minutes

Yields: 4 servings

Nutrition Facts: Calories: 323 | Carbs: 61g | Protein: 6g | Fat: 8g | Fiber: 5g

Ingredients:

- Two large eggs
- Two cups each of
    - Fresh pineapple, coarsely chopped
    - Old-fashioned rolled oats
    - Whole milk
- One cup of walnuts, chopped
- Half a cup of maple syrup
- One piece of ginger
- Two teaspoons of vanilla extract
- Half a teaspoon of salt

Method:

1. Preheat your oven to 400 degrees Fahrenheit.

2. Add the ginger, walnuts, pineapple, oats, and salt in a large bowl and mix them together. Add the mixture evenly among four ten-ounce ramekins and keep them aside.

3. Whisk the eggs along with the milk, maple syrup, and vanilla extract in a medium-sized bowl. Pour one-quarter of this mixture into each ramekin containing the oat-pineapple mixture.

4. Keep the ramekins on the baking sheet and bake them in the oven for about twenty-five minutes until the oats turn light golden brown on the top and have set properly.

5. Serve with some additional maple syrup on the side.

Caprese Salad

Total Prep & Cooking Time: 15 minutes

Yields: 4 servings

Nutrition Facts: Calories: 216 | Carbs: 4g | Protein: 13g | Fat: 16g | Fiber: 1g

Ingredients:

For the salad,

- Nine basil leaves (medium-sized)
- Eight ounces of fresh whole-milk mozzarella cheese
- Two tomatoes (medium-sized)
- One-fourth of a teaspoon of black pepper, freshly ground
- Half a teaspoon of Kosher salt, or one-fourth of a teaspoon of sea salt

For the dressing,

- One teaspoon of Dijon mustard
- One tablespoon each of
  - Balsamic vinegar
  - Olive oil

Method:

1. Add the olive oil, balsamic vinegar, and Dijon mustard into a small bowl and whisk them together with the help of a small hand whisk so that you get a smooth salad dressing. Keep it aside.

2. Cut the tomatoes into thin slices and try to get ten slices in total.

3. Cut the mozzarella into nine thin slices with the help of a sharp knife.

4. Place the slices of tomatoes and mozzarella on a serving plate, alternating and overlapping one another. Then, add the basil leaves on the top.

5. Season the salad with black pepper and salt and drizzle the prepared dressing on top.

6. Serve immediately.

One-Pot Chicken Soup

Total Prep & Cooking Time: 30 minutes

Yields: 6 servings

Nutrition Facts: Calories: 201 | Carbs: 20g | Protein: 16g | Fat: 7g | Fiber: 16g

Ingredients:

- Three cups of loosely packed chopped kale (or other greens of your choice)
- Two cups of chicken, shredded
- One can of white beans (about fifteen ounces), slightly drained
- Eight cups of broth (vegetable broth or chicken broth)
- Four cloves of garlic, minced
- One cup of yellow or white onion, diced
- One tablespoon of avocado oil (skip if you are using bacon)
- One strip of uncured bacon, chopped (optional)
- Black pepper + sea salt, according to taste

Method:

1. Place a Dutch oven or a large pot over medium heat. When it gets hot, add in the oil or bacon (optional), stirring occasionally, and allow it to get hot for about a minute.

2. Then, add in the diced onion and sauté for four to five minutes, occasionally stirring so that the onions get fragrant and translucent. Add in the minced garlic next and sauté for another two to three minutes. Be careful so as not to burn the ingredients.

3. Then, add the chicken, slightly drained white beans, and broth and bring the mixture to a simmer. Cook for about ten minutes to bring out all the flavors. Taste the mixture and add salt and pepper to season according to your preference. Add in the chopped kale in the last few minutes of cooking. Cover the pot and let it cook until the kale has wilted.

4. Serve hot.

Notes: *You can store any leftovers in the freezer for up to a month. Or, you can store them in the refrigerator for a maximum of three to four days. Simply reheat on the stovetop or in the microwave and eat it later.*

Chocolate Pomegranate Truffles

Total Prep & Cooking Time: 10 minutes

Yields: Twelve to Fourteen truffles

Nutrition Facts: Calories: 95 | Carbs: 26g | Protein: 1g | Fat: 2g | Fiber: 3g

Ingredients:

- One-third of a cup of pomegranate arils
- Half a teaspoon each of
  - Vanilla extract
  - Ground cinnamon
- Half a cup of ground flax seed
- Two tablespoons of cocoa powder (unsweetened)
- About one tablespoon of water
- One and a half cups of pitted Medjool dates
- One-eighth of a teaspoon of salt

Method:

1. Add the pitted dates in a food processor and blend until it begins to form a ball. Add some water and pulse again. Add in the vanilla, cinnamon, flax seeds, cocoa powder, and salt and blend until everything is combined properly.

2. Turn off the food processor and unplug it. Add in the pomegranate arils and fold them in the mixture so that they are distributed evenly.

3. Make twelve to fourteen balls using the mixture. You can create an outer coating or topping if you want by rolling the balls in finely shredded coconut or cocoa powder.

Notes: *You can store the chocolate pomegranate truffles in the fridge in an air-tight container for a maximum of three days.*

PART II

Are you worried that your hormones are not at their optimal levels? Here is a diet that will solve your problems.

Chapter 1: Health Benefits of the Hormone Diet

When it comes to getting healthy through weight loss, there's never any shortage of fitness crazes and diets that claim to have the secret to easy and sustainable weight loss. One of the latest diet plans that have come into the spotlight is the hormone diet, which claims that people often struggle to lose weight because of their hormones.

A hormone diet is a 3-step process that spans over six weeks and is designed to synchronize your hormones and promote a healthy body through detoxification, nutritional supplements, exercise, and diet. The diet controls what you eat and informs you about the correct time to eat to ensure maximum benefits to your hormones. Many books have been written on this topic with supporters of the diet assuring people that they can lose weight quickly and significantly through diet and exercise and reset or manipulate their hormones. Although the diet has a few variations, the central idea around each is that correcting the body's perceived hormonal imbalances is the key to losing weight.

The most important benefit of a hormone diet is that it takes a solid stance on improving overall health through weight loss and promoting regular exercise as well as natural, nutritious foods. Apart from that, it also focuses on adequate sleep, stress management, emotional health, and other healthy lifestyle habits that are all essential components that people should follow, whether it's a part of a diet or not. Including a water diet, it aims towards losing about twelve pounds in the 1st phase and 2 pounds a week after that.

Hormones have an essential role in the body's everyday processes, like helping bones grow, digesting food, etc. They act as "chemical messengers," instructing the cells to perform specific actions and are transported around the body through the bloodstream.

One of the very important food items to be included in the hormone diet is salmon. Salmon is rich in omega-3 fatty acids, Docosahexaenoic acid, and Eicosapentaenoic acid (EPA). It is rich in selenium too. These help to lower your blood pressure and also reduce the level of unhealthy cholesterol in the blood. These make you less prone to heart diseases. Salmon is a rich source of healthy fat. If consumed in sufficient amounts, it provides you energy and helps you get rid of unwanted body fat. Salmon is well-known for giving fantastic weight loss results as it has less saturated fat, unlike other protein sources. Salmon is packed with vitamins like vitamin-k, E, D, and A. These are extremely helpful for your eyes, bone joints, etc. These vitamins are also good for your brain, regulation of metabolic balance, and repairing your muscles. Salmon's vitamins and omega-3 fatty acids are amazing for sharpening your mind. It also improves your memory retention power. If you consume salmon, you are less likely to develop dementia or mental dis-functions. Salmon has anti-inflammatory properties and is low in omega-6 fatty acid content (which is pro-inflammatory in nature and is present in a huge amount in the modern diet). It promotes healthy skin and gives you radiant and glowing skin. It is good for the winter because it helps you to stay warm. It also provides lubrication to your joints because of the abundant presence of essential minerals and fatty acids in it. Apart from this, some other things to include in your diet are arugula, kale, ginger, avocado, carrots, and so on.

There are almost sixteen hormones that can influence weight. For example, the hormone leptin produced by your fat cells is considered a "satiety hormone," which makes you feel full by reducing your appetite. As a signaling hormone, it communicates with the part of your brain (hypothalamus) that controls food intake and appetite. Leptin informs the brain when there is enough fat in storage, and extra fat is not required. This helps prevent overeating. Individuals who are obese or overweight generally have very high levels of leptin in their blood. Research shows that the level of leptin in obese individuals was almost four times higher than that in individuals with normal weight.

Studies have found that fat hormones like leptin and adiponectin can promote long-term weight loss by reducing appetite and increasing metabolism. It is believed that both these fat hormones follow the same pathway in the brain to manage blood sugar (glucose) and body weight (Robert V. Considine, 1996).

Simply put, the hormone diet works by helping to create a calorie deficit through better nutritional habits and exercise, which ultimately results in weight loss. It's also essential to consult a doctor before following this detox diet or consuming any dietary supplements.

Chapter 2: Hormone-Rebalancing Smoothies

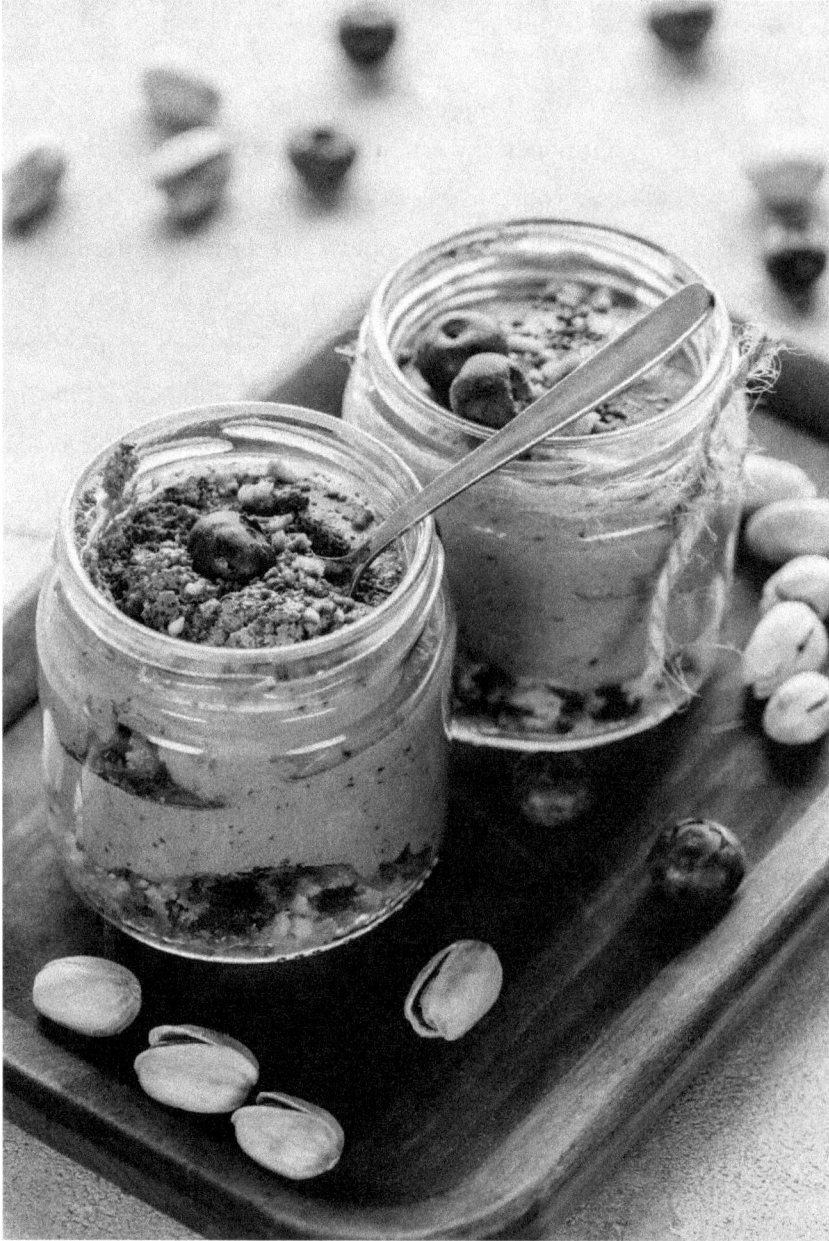

Estrogen Detox Smoothie

Total Prep & Cooking Time: 5 minutes

Yields: One glass

Nutrition Facts: Calories: 312 | Carbs: 47.9g | Protein: 18.6g | Fat: 8.5g | Fiber: 3g

Ingredients:

- Half a cup of hemp seeds
- Two kiwis (medium-sized)
- A quarter each of
  o Avocado (medium-sized)
  o Cucumber (medium-sized)
- Half a unit each of
  o Lemon (squeezed freshly)
  o Green apple
- One celery (medium-sized)
- A quarter cup of cilantro
- Two tbsps. of chis seeds
- Two cups of water (filtered)
- One tsp. of cacao nibs
- One tbsp. of coconut oil

Method:

1. Blend the ingredients all together to form a smoothie at high speed. The thickness can be adjusted according to your preference by adding more water to the mixture.

2. Serve and enjoy.

Dopamine Delight Smoothie

Total Prep Time: 10 minutes

Yields: One serving

Nutrition Facts: Calories: 383 | Carbs: 31g | Protein: 24g | Fat: 18.g | Fiber: 3g

Ingredients:

- Half a teaspoon of cinnamon (ground)
- Half a cup of peeled banana (the bananas must be frozen)
- One organic espresso, double shot (measuring half a cup)
- One tablespoon of chia seeds
- A three-fourth cup of soy milk (plain or vanilla-flavored)
- Protein powder, a serving (from the whey with the flavor of vanilla)

Method:

1. Fill in the bowl of your blender with all the ingredients (from the section of ingredients) except the whey protein powder and then proceed by switching to a high-speed blending option. Make sure it acquires a smooth consistency and then pour it out.

2. Now you may add the protein powder and give it another shot of blend until the whole things get incorporated, a bit of the goat cheese (already crumbled).

Breakfast Smoothie Bowl

Total Prep Time: 10 minutes

Yields: 2 servings

Nutrition Facts: Calories: 290 | Carbs: 53g | Protein: 6g | Fat: 8g | Fiber: 9g

Ingredients:

- One cup of thoroughly rinsed blueberries (fresh and ripe)
- A sundry of nuts and fruits for garnishing, which includes – strawberries, bananas (thinly sliced), peanuts (Spanish), kiwi (chopped), segments of tangerine, and raspberries.
- One cup of Greek yogurt

For the preparation of honey flax granola,

- Two tablespoons each of
  - Flaxseeds
  - Vegetable oil
- Oats (old-fashioned), approximately a cup
- One tablespoon of honey

Method:

1. Set your oven at a temperature of 350 degrees F.

2. Preparation of the smoothie: collect the diverse types of berries, wash them thoroughly, and then put them in the blender and turn it on. Make an even mixture out of it. Add some amount of the yogurt and blend it again to form a smooth texture.

3. For preparing the granola: Take a small-sized bowl and then drizzle a few drops oil in it. Then add the oats, flax, and honey to the oil, one by one, and mix it well. You are required to toss the bowl thoroughly to get the mixture well-coated with the poured oil. After you are done, place the oats mixture in a baking sheet evenly. Bake it for about twenty minutes. This mark will be enough to give the oats a beautiful tinge of golden brown. Allow it to cool.

4. Now you will require a shallow bowl to spoon in some yogurt, and this will be the first layer. Form a second layer with the various fruits and nuts and finally for the third layer, top with the granola.

5. Enjoy.

Notes:

- *Using frozen nuts and fruits in a warm-weather will get much to your relief.*

- *For a vegan smoothie bowl, sub the yogurt with coconut or almond yogurt.*

- *Give the pan a few strokes while baking the oats.*

Blueberry Detox Smoothie

Total Prep Time: Ten minutes

Yields: One serving

Nutrition Facts: Calories: 326 | Carbs: 65g | Protein: 4g | Fat: 8g | Fiber: 9g

Ingredients:

- One cup of wild blueberries (frozen)
- One banana (sliced into several pieces) frozen
- Orange juice (approximately half a cup)
- Cilantro leaves, fresh (approximately a measuring a small handful size)
- A quarter of an entire avocado
- A quarter cup of water

Method:

1. Add cilantro, avocado, water, blueberries, banana, and orange juice in the blender and then process.

2. Make the ingredients integrated so well that they become smooth in their consistency.

Notes: *It is recommended that you add the potent herb, cilantro, or parsley in a small amount when consuming this smoothie for the first time, as it might trigger a mild headache. If you do not get a headache, you may add a bit more of the cilantro leaves.*

Maca Mango Smoothie

Total Prep & Cooking Time: 2 minutes

Yields: 2 servings

Nutrition Facts: Calories: 53 | Carbs: 13g | Protein: 1g | Fat: 3g | Fiber: 1.5g

Ingredients:

- One and a half cups each of
    - Fresh mango
    - Frozen mango
- One tablespoon each of
    - Ground flaxseed
    - Nut butter
- One teaspoon of ground turmeric
- Two teaspoons of maca root powder
- Three-quarter cups of nut milk
- One frozen banana

Method:

1. Blend all the ingredients together to get a smooth mixture.

2. Adjust consistency by adding nut milk.

3. Once done, divide into two glasses and enjoy!

Pituitary Relief Smoothie

Total Prep & Cooking Time: 5 minutes

Yields: 2 servings

Nutrition Facts: Calories: 174 | Carbs: 18.3g | Protein: 9.7g | Fat: 8.3g | Fiber: 14.4g

Ingredients:

- One teaspoon of coconut oil
- One fresh or frozen ripe banana
- One tablespoon of raw sesame seeds
- Two teaspoons each of
  o Chia seeds
  o Raw Maca powder
  o Raw Spirulina
- Two cups of water
- Two tablespoons of hulled hemp seeds

Method:

1. You have to use a blender to process this smoothie. Add the hulled hemp seeds, sesame seeds, and water in the blender and process them. Do it at high speed, and it will only require a minute. This will give you raw-milk like texture.

2. Then, add the following ingredients into it – coconut oil, banana, chia seeds, Maca, and Spirulina, and process the ingredients once again but this time on medium speed for another minute or so. Everything will become well incorporated.

3. You have to drink this smoothie on an empty stomach.

Notes: *In order to make the smoothie rich in antioxidants, you can add some fresh fruits like blueberries, kiwi, and raspberries.*

Chapter 2: Easy Breakfast Recipes

Scrambled Eggs With Feta and Tomatoes

Total Prep & Cooking Time: 10 minutes

Yields: One Plate

Nutrition Facts: Calories: 421 | Carbs: 8.6g | Protein: 20.3g | Fat: 35.1g | Fiber: 1.6g

Ingredients:

- One tbsp. each of
  - o Olive oil (extra virgin)
  - o Freshly chopped parsley, basil, dill or chives
- Half a cup of cherry tomatoes (each tomato sliced into half)
- Two ounces of crumbled feta cheese (approximately a quarter cup)
- Two eggs are beaten
- Two tbsp. of onion (diced)
- To taste:
  - o Black pepper
  - o Kosher salt

Method:

1. Keep the beaten eggs in a small-sized bowl and then season it with a pinch of pepper and salt. Set the bowl aside.

2. Use a nonstick skillet to proceed with the cooking. Pour two tbsp. of olive oil. Then add the diced onions. Stir over moderate heat and cook until softened. Make sure that the onions do not look brown. This process should get done by a minute.

3. Add half a cup of tomatoes to skillet and then continue to mix for about two minutes.

4. Now you may add the eggs. Using a spatula, gather the beaten eggs to the center by moving spatula all over the skillet.

5. The eggs will take an additional minute to get cooked. So after that mark, add the parsley or other herbs (if preferred) and feta cheese. Keep the eggs underdone as they will get cooked completely after they are served in the plate itself (from the residual heat). Therefore, cook the entire thing in the skillet for 30 seconds only.

6. Take a serving plate and transfer the eggs to it. Top with some sprinkled parsley and feta cheese, drizzled with some oil, and seasoned with some pepper and salt. These additions are optional and may vary as per your desire.

Smashed Avo and Quinoa

Total Prep & Cooking Time: 15 minutes

Yields: Six bowls

Nutrition Facts: Calories: 492 | Carbs: 67g | Protein: 15g | Fat: 20g | Fiber: 13g

Ingredients:

- One avocado skinned, cut into half, and then pitted
- A handful of cilantro or coriander
- Half a lemon (juiced)
- A quarter red onion (diced finely)
- One-eighth teaspoon of cayenne pepper
- To taste: Sea salt

For the Greens,

- One handful of kale
- One handful of soft herbs (basil, parsley or mint)
- One handful of chard or spinach
- For frying: butter or coconut oil

Serve with,

- One cup of quinoa (cooked)

Method:

1. You will require a frying pan to get this done. To it, add the coconut oil or butter (whichever you prefer) and add the greens. Toss them carefully and then sauté over moderate heat. Stop when they become soft.

2. Mix the onion, cayenne, avocado, cilantro, salt, lemon, and pepper to a bowl and mix them completely. The pepper and salt must be added according to the taste.

3. Add cooked quinoa to the tossed greens and heat altogether over low heat.

4. Take a serving plate and place the quinoa mixture and greens to it. Crown the whole thing with smashed avocado and then serve.

Hormone Balancing Granola

Total Prep & Cooking Time: 35 minutes

Yields: 8 servings

Nutrition Facts: Calories: 360 | Carbs: 19.8g | Protein: 5.1g | Fat: 28.8g | Fiber: 5.8g

Ingredients:

- One-third cup each of
  - Flaxseed meal
  - Pumpkin seeds
  - Seedless raisins
- Two teaspoons of cinnamon
- One teaspoon of vanilla extract
- Four tablespoons of maple syrup
- Five tablespoons of melted coconut oil
- A quarter cup of unsweetened coconut flakes
- Two-thirds cup each of
  - Chopped pecans
  - Chopped brazil nuts
- Two tablespoons of ground chia seeds

Method:

1. Set the temperature of the oven to 180 degrees F and preheat.

2. In a food processor, chop the pecans and the Brazil nuts. Then, mix these chopped nuts with coconut flakes, seeds, and other nuts present in the list of ingredients.

3. Add maple syrup, coconut oil, cinnamon, and vanilla extract in a separate bowl and combine well.

4. Now, take the wet ingredients and pour them into the dry ingredients. Mix thoroughly so that everything has become coated properly.

5. Place the prepared mixture in the oven for half an hour and cook.

6. Once done, cut into pieces and serve.

Chapter 3: Healthy Lunch Recipes

Easy Shakshuka

Total Prep & Cooking Time: 30 minutes

Yields: Six servings

Nutrition Facts: Calories: 154 | Carbs: 4.1g | Protein: 9g | Fat: 7.8g | Fiber: 0g

Ingredients:

- Olive oil (extra virgin)
- Two chopped green peppers
- One teaspoon each of
  - Paprika (sweet)
  - Coriander (ground)
- A pinch of red pepper (flakes)
- Half a cup of tomato sauce
- A quarter cup each of
  - Mint leaves (freshly chopped)
  - Parsley leaves (chopped freshly)
- One yellow onion, large-sized (chopped)
- Two cloves of garlic, chopped
- Half a teaspoon of cumin (ground)
- Six cups of chopped tomatoes (Vine-ripe)
- Six large-sized eggs
- To taste: Pepper and salt

Method:

1. You will require a large-sized skillet (made of cast iron). Pour three tablespoons of oil and heat it. After bringing the oil to boil, add the peppers, spices, onions, garlic, pepper, and salt. Stir time to time to cook the veggies for five minutes until they become softened.

2. After the vegetables become soft, add the chopped tomatoes and then tomato sauce. Cover the skillet and simmer for an additional fifteen minutes.

3. Now, you may remove the lid from the pan and then cook a touch more to thicken the consistency. At this point, you may adjust the taste.

4. Make six cavities within the tomato mixture and crack one egg each inside the cavities.

5. Cover the skillet after reducing the heat and allow it to cook so that the eggs settle into the cavities.

6. Keep track of the time and accordingly uncover the skillet and then add mint and parsley. Season with more black and red pepper according to your desire. Serve them warm with the sort of bread you wish.

Ginger Chicken

Total Prep & Cooking Time: 50 minutes

Yields: Six Servings

Nutrition Facts: Calories: 310 | Carbs: 6g | Protein: 37g | Fat: 16g | Fiber: 1g

Ingredients:

- A one-kilogram pack of chicken thighs (skinless and boneless)
- Four cloves of garlic (chopped finely)
- A fifteen-gram pack of coriander (fresh and chopped)
- Two tablespoons of sunflower oil
- One teaspoon each of
  o Turmeric (ground)
  o Chili powder (mild)
- A four hundred milliliter can of coconut milk (reduced-fat)
- One cube of chicken stock
- One ginger properly peeled and chopped finely (it should be of the size of a thumb)
- One lime, juiced
- Two medium-sized onions
- One red chili, sliced and the seeds removed (fresh)

Method:

1. Make the chicken thighs into three large chunks and marinate them with chili powder, garlic, coriander (half of the entire amount), ginger, oil (one tbsp.), and lime juice. Cover the bowl after stirring them well and then store it in the fridge until oven-ready.

2. Marinade the chicken and keep overnight for better flavor.

3. Chop the onions finely (it is going to be the simplest for preparing the curry) before dropping them into the food processor. Pour oil into the frying pan (large-sized) and heat it. Then add chopped onions and stir them thoroughly for eight minutes until the pieces become soft. Then pour the turmeric powder and stir for an additional minute.

4. Now add the chicken mixture and cook on high heat until you notice a change in its color. Pour the chicken stock, chili, and coconut milk and after covering the pan simmer for another twenty minutes. Sprinkle the left-over coriander leaves and then serve hot.

5. Enjoy.

Carrot and Miso Soup

Total Prep & Cooking Time: 1 hour

Yields: Four bowls of soup

Nutrition Facts: Calories: 76 | Carbs: 8.76g | Protein: 4.83g | Fat: 2.44g | Fiber: 1.5g

Ingredients:

- Two tbsps. of oil
- Garlic, minced (four cloves)
- One inch of garlic (grated)
- Three tbsps. of miso paste (white)
- One diced onion
- One pound of carrot (sliced thinly)
- Four cups of vegetable stock
- To taste: Pepper and Salt

For garnishing,

- Two scallions (sliced thinly)
- Chili pepper (seven spices)
- One nori roasted (make thin slivers)
- Sesame oil

Method:

1. Using a soup pot will be convenient to proceed with. Pour oil in a pot and then heat over a high flame. Now you may put garlic, carrot, and onion and sauté them thoroughly. Cook for about ten minutes so that the onions turn translucent.

2. Then add the ginger and vegetable stock. Mix them well and cook all together. Put the flame to simmer. Cover the pot while cooking to make the carrot tender. This will take another thirty minutes.

3. Put off the flame and puree the soup with the help of an immersion blender.

4. Use a small-sized bowl to whisk together a spoonful of the soup and the white miso paste. Stir until the paste dissolve and pour the mixture back to the pot.

5. Add pepper and salt if required.

6. Divide the soup among four bowls and enrich its feel by adding scallions, sesame oil, seven spices, and nori.

Arugula Salad

Total Prep & Cooking Time: 1 hour 10 minutes

Yields: Two bowls of salad

Nutrition Facts: Calories: 336.8 | Carbs: 30.6g | Protein: 7.7g | Fat: 22.2g | Fiber: 7.3g

Ingredients:

For the salad,

- Two medium-sized beets (boiled or roasted for about an hour), skinned and sliced into pieces that can easily be bitten
- Four tablespoons of goat cheese
- Approximately 2.5 oz. of baby arugula (fresh)
- A quarter cup of walnuts (chopped roughly before toasting)

For the dressing,

- Three tablespoons of olive oil (extra virgin)
- A quarter tsp. each of
  - Mustard powder (dried)
  - Pepper
- Half a tsp. each of
  - Salt
  - Sugar

- One and a half tablespoons of lemon juice

Method:

1. For preparing the vinaigrette, place all the ingredients (listed in the dressing ingredients section) in a jar and then shake them to emulsify. At this stage, before starting with the process of emulsification, you may add or remove the ingredients as per your liking.

2. Get the salad assembled (again depending upon the taste you want to give it), add a fistful of arugula leaves, place some chopped beets (after they have been cooked), and finally the toasted walnuts (already chopped).

3. Drizzle vinaigrette over the salad and enjoy.

Notes:

- *Coat the beets with oil (olive), roll them up in an aluminum foil, and then roast the beets at a temperature of 400 degrees F.*

- *And for boiling the beets, immerse them in water after transferring to a pot and simmer them for 45 minutes.*

Kale Soup

Total Prep & Cooking Time: 55 minutes

Yields: 8 servings

Nutrition Facts: Calories: 277.3 | Carbs: 50.9g | Protein: 9.6g | Fat: 4.5g | Fiber: 10.3g

Ingredients:

- Two tbsps. of dried parsley
- One tbsp. of Italian seasoning
- Salt and pepper
- Thirty oz. of drained cannellini beans
- Six peeled and cubed white potatoes
- Fifteen ounces of diced tomatoes
- Six vegetable Bouillon cubes
- Eight cups of water
- One bunch of kale (with chopped leaves and stems removed)
- Two tbsps. of chopped garlic
- One chopped yellow onion
- Two tbsps. of olive oil

Method:

1. At first, take a large soup pot, add in some olive oil, and heat it.

2. Add garlic and onion. Cook them until soft.

3. Then stir in the kale and cook for about two minutes, until wilted.

4. Pour the water and add the beans, potatoes, tomatoes, vegetable bouillon, parsley, and the Italian seasoning.

5. On medium heat, simmer the soup for about twenty-five minutes, until the potatoes are cooked through.

6. Finally, do the seasoning with salt and pepper according to your taste.

Roasted Sardines

Total Prep & Cooking Time: 25 minutes

Yields: 4 servings

Nutrition Facts: Calories: 418 | Carbs: 2.6g | Protein: 41g | Fat: 27.2g | Fiber: 0.8g

Ingredients:

- 3.5 oz. of cherry tomatoes (cut them in halves)
- One medium-sized red onion (chopped finely)
- Two tablespoons each of
  o   Chopped parsley
  o   Extra-virgin olive oil
- One clove of garlic (halved)
- Eight units of fresh sardines (gutted and cleaned, heads should be cleaned)
- A quarter teaspoon of chili flakes
- One teaspoon of toasted cumin seeds
- Half a lemon (zested and juiced)

Method:

1. Set the temperature of the oven to 180 degrees C and preheat. Take a roasting tray and grease it lightly.

2. Take a bowl and add the tomatoes and onions in it. Add the lemon juice too and toss the veggies in the lemon juice. Now, add the zest, olive oil, chili, cumin, garlic, and parsley and toss everything once again.

3. Use pepper and salt to season the mixture. The cavity of the sardines has to be filled. Use some of the tomato and onion mixture for this purpose. Once done, place the sardines on the prepared roasting tray. Take the remaining mixture and scatter it over the sardines.

4. Roast the sardines for about 10-15 minutes, and by the end of this, they should be cooked thoroughly.

5. Serve and enjoy!

Chapter 4: Tasty Dinner Recipes

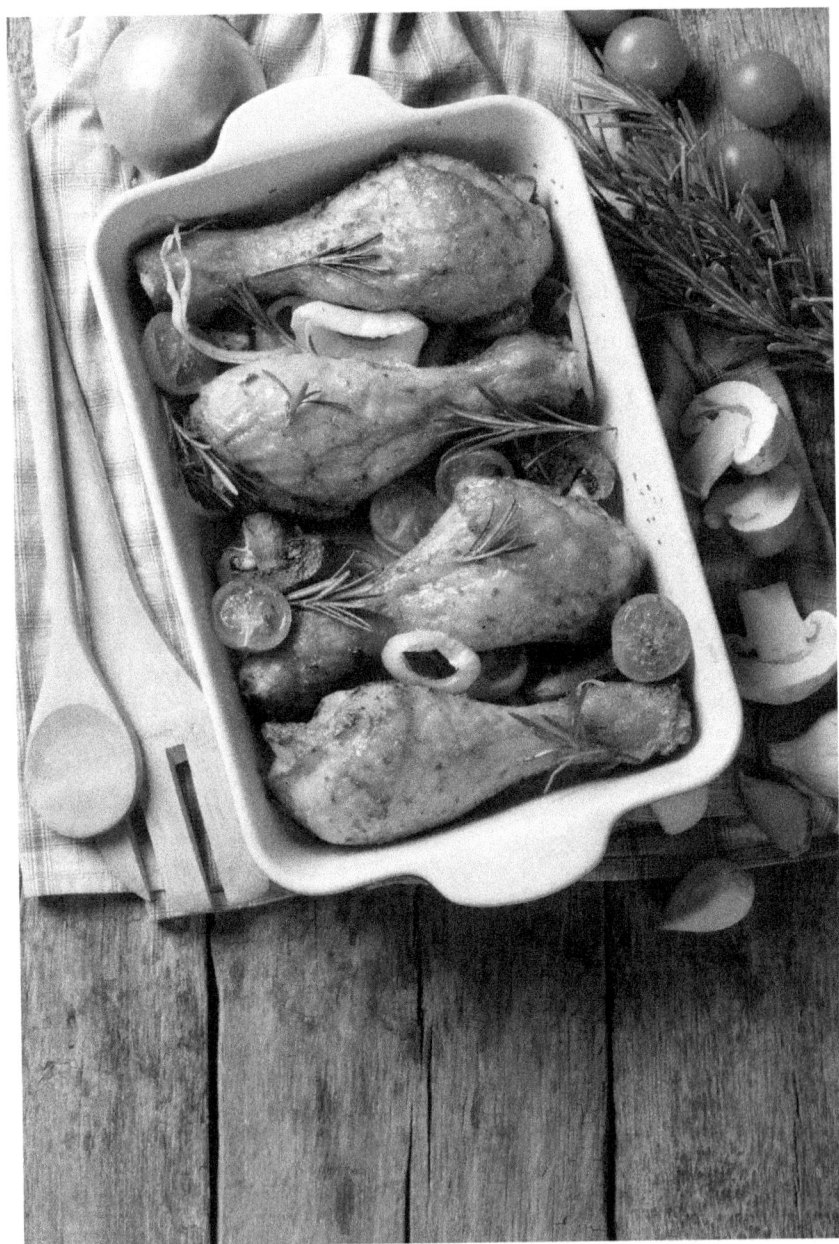

Rosemary Chicken

Total Prep & Cooking Time: 50 minutes

Yields: 4 servings

Nutrition Facts: Calories: 232 | Carbs: 3.9g | Protein: 26.7g | Fat: 11.6g | Fiber: 0.3g

Ingredients:

- Four chicken breast halves (skinless and boneless)
- One-eighth tsp. kosher salt
- One-fourth tsp. ground black pepper
- One and a half tbsps. of lemon juice
- One and a half tbsps. of Dijon mustard
- Two tbsps. of freshly minced rosemary
- Three tbsps. of olive oil
- Eight minced garlic cloves

Method:

1. At first, preheat a grill to medium-high heat. The grate needs to be lightly oiled.

2. Take a bowl and add lemon juice, mustard, rosemary, olive oil, garlic, salt, and ground black pepper. Whisk them together.

3. Take a resealable plastic bag and place the chicken breasts in it. Over the chicken, pour the garlic mixture (reserve one-eighth cup of it).

4. Seal the bag and start massaging the marinade gently into the chicken. Allow it to stand for about thirty minutes at room temperature.

5. Then on the preheated grill, place the chicken and cook for about four minutes.

6. Flip the chicken and baste it with the marinade reserved and then cook for about five minutes, until thoroughly cooked.

Finally, cover it with a foil and allow it to rest for about 2 minutes before you serve them.

Corned Beef and Cabbage

Total Prep & Cooking Time: 2 hours 35 minutes

Yields: 5 servings

Nutrition Facts: Calories: 868.8 | Carbs: 75.8g | Protein: 50.2g | Fat: 41.5g | Fiber: 14g

Ingredients:

- One big cabbage head (cut it into small wedges)
- Five peeled carrots (chopped into three-inch pieces)
- Ten red potatoes (small)
- Three pounds of corned beef brisket (along with the packet of spice)

Method:

1. At first, in a Dutch oven or a large pot, place the corned beef, and cover it with water. Then add in the spices from the packet of spices that came along with the beef. Cover the pot, bring it to a boil, and finally reduce it to a simmer. Allow it to simmer for about 2 hours and 30 minutes or until tender.

2. Add carrots and whole potatoes, and cook them until the vegetables are tender. Add the cabbage wedges and cook for another fifteen minutes. Then finally remove the meat and allow it to rest for fifteen minutes.

3. Take a bowl, place the vegetables in it, and cover it. Add broth (which is reserved in the pot) as much as you want. Then finally cut the meat against the grain.

Roasted Parsnips and Carrots

Total Prep & Cooking Time: 1 hour

Yields: 4 servings

Nutrition Facts: Calories: 112 | Carbs: 27g | Protein: 2g | Fat: 1g | Fiber: 7g

Ingredients:

- Two tbsps. of freshly minced parsley or dill
- One and a half tsp. of freshly ground black pepper
- One tbsp. kosher salt
- Three tbsps. of olive oil
- One pound of unpeeled carrots
- Two pounds of peeled parsnips

Method:

1. At first, preheat your oven to 425 degrees.

2. If the carrots and parsnips are thick, then cut them into halves lengthwise.

3. Then, slice each of them diagonally into one inch thick slices. Don't cut them too small because the vegetables will anyway shrink while you cook them.

4. Take a sheet pan, and place the cut vegetables on it.

5. Then add some olive oil, pepper, salt, and toss them nicely.

6. Roast them for about twenty to forty minutes (the roasting time depends on the size of the vegetables), accompanied by occasional tossing. Continue to roast until the carrots and parsnips become tender.

7. Finally, sprinkle some dill and serve.

Herbed Salmon

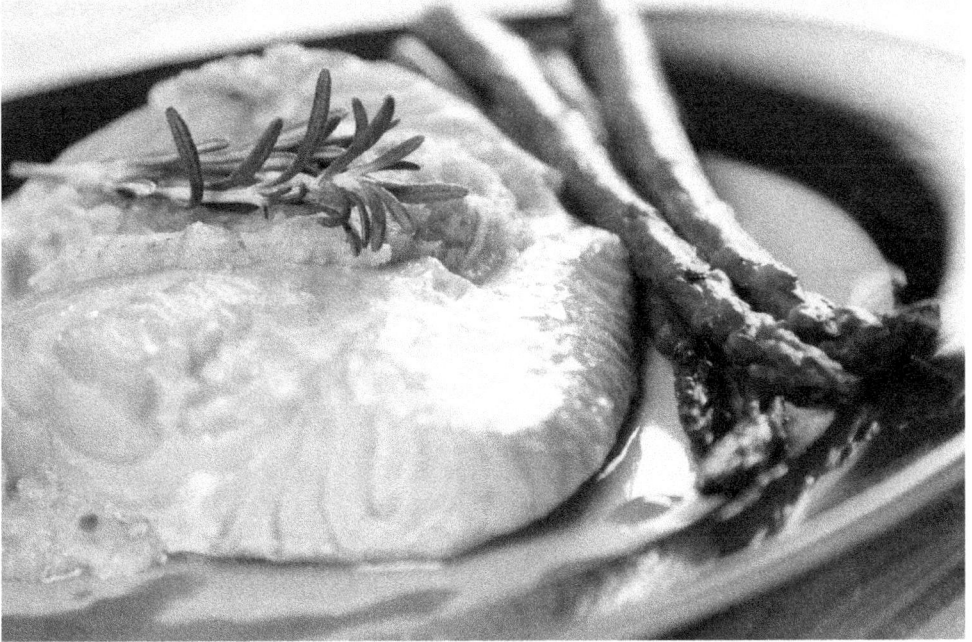

Total Prep & Cooking Time: 30 minutes

Yields: 4 servings

Nutrition Facts: Calories: 301 | Carbs: 1g | Protein: 29g | Fat: 19g | Fiber: 0g

Ingredients:

- Half a tsp. of dried thyme or two tsps. of freshly minced thyme
- Half a tsp. of pepper

- Three-fourth tsp. of salt

- One tbsp. of olive oil

- One tbsp. freshly minced rosemary or one tsp. of crushed dried rosemary.

- Four minced cloves of garlic

- Four (six ounces) fillets of salmon

Method:

1. At first, preheat your oven to 425 degrees.

2. Take a 15 by 10 by 1 inch baking pan and grease it.

3. Place the salmon on it while keeping the skin side down.

4. Combine the garlic cloves, rosemary, thyme, salt, and pepper. Spread it evenly over the salmon fillets.

5. Roast them for about fifteen to eighteen minutes until they reach your desired doneness.

Chipotle Cauliflower Tacos

Total Prep & Cooking Time: 30 minutes

Yields: 8 servings

Nutrition Facts: Calories: 440 | Carbs: 51.6g | Protein: 10.1g | Fat: 24g | Fiber: 9g

Ingredients:

For the tacos,

- Four tablespoons of avocado oil
- One head of cauliflower (large-sized, chopped into bite-sized florets)
- One cup of cilantro (freshly chopped)
- One tablespoon each of
  o Fresh lime juice
  o Maple syrup or honey
- Two tsps. of chipotle adobo sauce
- Cracked black pepper
- One teaspoon of salt
- 4-8 units of garlic cloves (freshly minced)

For the Chipotle Aioli,

- A quarter cup of chipotle adobo sauce
- Half a cup each of
  o Sour cream
  o Clean mayo

One teaspoon of sea salt

Two cloves of garlic (minced)

For serving,

- Almond flour tortillas
- Guacamole
- Almond ricotta cheese
- Sliced tomatoes, radish, and cabbage

Method:

1. Set the temperature of the oven to 425 degrees F. Now, use parchment paper to line a pan. Take the bite-sized florets of the cauliflower and spread them evenly on the pan. Use 2-4 tbsps. of avocado oil, pepper, salt, and minced garlic and drizzle it on the pan.

2. Roast the cauliflower for half an hour at 425 degrees F and halfway through the process, flip the florets.

3. When you are roasting the cauliflower, take the rest of the ingredients of the cauliflower and mix them in a bowl. Once everything has been properly incorporated, set the mixture aside.

4. Now, take another bowl and in it, add the ingredients of the chipotle aioli. Mix them and set the bowl aside.

5. If you have any other taco fixings, get them ready.

6. Once the cauliflower is ready, toss the florets in the chipotle sauce.

7. Serve the cauliflower in tortillas along with fixings of your choice and the chipotle aioli.

Be gentle with yourself throughout this process as it will be uncomfortable at times and will require strength. This book will help you through it, as you are not alone. I hope that this book also reminds you that many other people are suffering from the same type of food-related disorders as you are and that you are not alone in that either. This book will take a step-by-step approach, which will make for the highest chance of recovery. If at any time you need to take a break in order to think about the information you have learned, feel free to do so, but make sure you come back to this book quite soon after. Going through this process of recovery can be a lot, but with the right support, it will be possible.

You have already taken the first step in recovery, which is acknowledging that you have an issue. For that, I congratulate you!

PART III

Chapter 1: What is the Alkaline Diet?

We eat the foods that we eat for all kinds of different reasons. Sure, from an evolutionary standpoint, we eat food so that we can take in calories and convert them into energy in order to fuel our bodies and keep us going throughout the entire day. The food we eat also provides us with the essential nutrients that our bodies need in order to keep them running in an optimal manner.

But we also eat food for pleasure, the sheer joy of tasting something amazing that we truly love. We eat socially. Food has been a way of bringing people together since the very dawn of civilization. Sometimes we use food for comfort and sometimes we use it to mark formal and important occasions. We use food as a proving ground over which to test out new prospective romantic partners.

And yet, for all that food can do for us, so many of us take it for granted and don't seek out ways to make our food work for us. Used correctly, food and nutrition are tools that can turn our bodies into the healthiest and efficient powerhouse that nature intended them to be.

With so many different diets and nutrition plans out there, it can be hard to know which one is right for you. Well, you're reading this book so you already know that you're on the right track!

Indeed, the alkaline diet is a tried and tested way to get the most out of your body. But how does it work? Why does it work? How can eating an alkaline diet optimize your body and health?

The key to understanding the science and chemistry behind how the foods we eat affect us is to understand that just like the fundamental laws of physics, every action has an equal and opposite reaction. Or in other words, everything that we put into our bodies will affect us based on the characteristics of that particular food item. So if we eat a lot of things that cause the same or similar effects on our bodies, we can influence and even control the effects and changes that our body takes by carefully selecting the foods that we eat and what effect they have on our bodies. As the popular saying goes — you are what you eat.

To illustrate, imagine you are walking through the woods and you accidentally brush up against a poison ivy leaf. Well, sorry to say it, but there is a very good chance that you are going to develop an itchy poison ivy rash. If however, you get completely naked and roll around in an entire patch of poison ivy, you are pretty much guaranteed to get poison ivy and a whole lot of it!

Humorous examples aside, it stands to reason that if we know that a particular food or food group has a particular effect on our body, we can effectively control any number of internal body systems by carefully planning and selecting the foods we eat.

So how does the alkaline diet promote health? Well, the alkaline diet is all about balance. So many of the negative health issues in our lives are the result of an imbalance in our bodies. So much of the history of medicine revolves around finding the ideal balances for the human body.

For many, many years, doctors around the world attributed all of our health conditions, whether good or ill, to a balance or imbalance in what they referred to as the "humors". As far back as Ancient Greece and Ancient Rome, there was a near-universal belief that four humors or bodily fluids influenced every aspect of health and temperament, and ill health or ill temperament was the result of deficiencies or excesses on one or more of these four humors. These four humors were black bile, yellow bile, phlegm, and blood. Each of these four humors was associated with a particular personality type and other such characteristics.

When a person came to an ancient doctor with an ailment, the ancient doctor would examine their patient to determine their temperament and along with other factors would determine where their imbalance in humors was, and then they would come up with a treatment plan with the intention of balancing the patient's humors. So in other words, for millennia, the goal of medicine has been to achieve balance in the human body.

And while many of the theories and practices of ancient physicians have long ago fallen out of use in favor of new techniques and schools of thought, modern science has nevertheless confirmed at least some aspects of ancient medicine, namely, the concept of balance itself.

While we don't hear much about black bile, yellow bile, or phlegm anymore in modern medicine, the fourth humor that ancient doctors treated is certainly still extremely prominent in modern medicine — blood.

Blood is still very much our life force just as it was believed by ancient doctors. Blood is the fluid that keeps us living and breathing and a proper medical understanding is absolutely integral to maintain overall good health.

So how can we maintain a good balance in our blood? What aspect of our blood do we even need to balance? What negative effects can we avoid by maintaining balanced blood and what positive ones can we promote?

While those ancient doctors were certainly on the right track, they had a few key factors wrong so, in order to move forward, we are going to need a firmer and more modern grasp of the science behind our health and nutrition.

To understand this concept a little bit better, we need to understand one of the most fundamental aspects of chemistry. This integral part of chemistry and science as a whole is known as the pH balance or the pH scale. We are going to learn all about the pH balance or the pH scale and how it can affect our bodies in a positive way in the following chapters. First, we will learn what a pH balance is.

Chapter 2: What is a pH Balance?

The first thing we need to understand on our journey to the perfect internal balance via the alkaline diet is exactly just what the pH balance is. Furthermore, we need to understand how the chemical characteristics of a substance or fluid play a role in determining where it falls on the pH scale.

What exactly does the pH scale measure? In short, the pH scale is a measure of the acidity or basicity of solution in which the solvent is water. Such a solution is known as an aqueous solution. In other words, when a substance is dissolved in or is otherwise mixed with water, it can then be tested and measured on the pH scale.

An aqueous solution can be defined as either an acid or a base, as this is precisely what the pH scale is meant to determine. An aqueous solution that is basic is referred to as being alkaline. This gives us a pretty good indication of what the alkaline diet is all about. The pH scale itself is a type of scale known as a logarithmic scale. This means that each equidistant quantified measure is an order of magnitude greater than the previous measurement on the scale. The scale ranges from zero to fourteen, with a neutral pH value being in the middle at seven.

Solutions that have a pH value of less the median value of seven are defined as being acidic, while the opposite scenario, in which a solution is measured to have a pH value of higher than seven — that solution is called basic. Water that is pure and unadulterated is pH neutral which is to say that it should prove to have a pH value of seven when tested, as natural dihydrogen oxide, the chemical name for water is neither a base nor an acid. If that is not the case, then the water should be tested for impurities.

While it is possible for an aqueous solution to have a pH value greater than fourteen or less than zero, these would have to be extremely acidic or extremely basic solutions and would not only be decisively deadly to ingest and even extremely dangerous just to touch. Therefore, for practical purposes, official pH values are nearly always represented on a scale between zero and fourteen.

The pH scale is defined by a set of international standards that are determined and agreed upon by an international scientific body. There are several ways to test the pH level of an aqueous solution, with one of the most notable ones being the use of a glass electrode combined with a pH meter. This scientific instrument determines the difference between a pH electrode and a control electrode in terms of their respective electrical potential. This difference in the electrical potential of a solution relates directly to the acidity of the solution and can therefore be used to give it a standard value.

Another very popular and frequently used means by which to test the pH value of an aqueous solution is by using one of the various compounds known as pH indicators.

A pH indicator is generally some kind of substance that when mixed with an aqueous solution results in a chemical reaction that will literally change the color of the solution, and by examining and comparing the color of the resulting solution, the pH value of the solution can be determined. There are other pH indicators that indicate the pH level of a solution by chemical reactions that result in other physical indicators such as odor for example. However, by far the most common variety of pH indicators are visual in nature, generally based around color.

One of the most common types of pH indicators is the naturally occurring family of chemical compounds called anthocyanin. These compounds naturally change color reflects the pH balance of whatever item the compound is found within. Generally, these compounds are found in colored plant leaves or other plant parts. One of the most common sources of these pH indicating compounds is from the leaves of a red cabbage. The reason for this is because it is quite easy to extract anthocyanin from a red cabbage making it the perfect resource for a homemade pH indicator test for either health or educational purposes.

Anthocyanin can be found in many different plants though, such as the leaves of the aforementioned red cabbage, but also in certain flowers such as the geranium, the poppy, and also rose petals. Berries and stems can also house anthocyanin compounds such as blueberries and blackcurrants as well as rhubarb. In short, most plants or vegetables that have reddish, purplish, or bluish color in all likelihood contain at least a small amount of anthocyanin compound. When used as a pH indicator by mixing it with an aqueous solution, an anthocyanin compound will become redder the more acidic the solution is and will turn from red to purple to blue the more alkaline the solution is.

Another very commonly used pH indicator since medieval times is the substance called litmus which is derived from various species of lichen. In fact, the word litmus itself means colored moss in its original language, Old Norse. Just like anthocyanin compounds, litmus will turn red when exposed to acidic solutions and blue when exposed to basic solutions. You may even be familiar with the term 'litmus test'. It has come to be used very commonly and very broadly as a metaphor for anything that could be used to soundly distinguish between multiple options.

So with pH balance being fundamental to the chemical nature of all kinds of biological material including the foods we eat, how do we know if and how such foods are affecting our health? We will continue learning about pH imbalance in our bodies to find out. The next chapter will go into the science of how pH balance or more specifically imbalance can affect our bodies and our health.

Chapter 3: The Science Behind pH Imbalance

Every single substance in the world has a pH balance and that includes all of us. Sure, we don't make cabbages change color when we pick them up, but our bodies must maintain a certain pH level in order to live and function properly. This pH balance that is naturally maintained in our bodies is called the acid-based balance and it is quite literally exactly what it sounds like — the balance of acidic and basic substances in your body. More specifically though, when we are referring to the acid-base balance of our bodies, we are most often referring to the pH balance of our blood.

The human body is designed with a few systems in place intended to keep the natural pH levels regulated at an appropriate balance between acidity and alkalinity. Both the kidneys as well as the lungs have a very important role to play in this process. As we previously laid out, the pH balance is generally expressed as a value between zero and fourteen, with seven being the neutral value. And remember that pure and unadulterated water should have a pH value of exactly seven. Knowing then that water is neutral seven on the pH scale, and knowing also that our bodies are designed to maintain an even pH balance, it would stand to reason that our blood should have a neutral pH value of seven as well, right?

Well, not quite. And this is a major key to understand the alkaline diet. The ideal blood pH level is not actually a neutral seven but instead generally should be about a 7.40 on the pH scale. This value can vary slightly from person to person, but that is the standard average. And yes, that's right— the human body should have a blood pH level that is a little bit on the alkaline side.

Generally speaking, it is the kidneys and lungs that regulate this pH level, so if they are not functioning normally, the blood pH level can become imbalanced. This kind of pH imbalance can lead to serious medical conditions which are called acidosis or alkalosis depending on which direction the imbalance goes in. It is important to note that these serious medical conditions must be treated by a medical professional and diet alone cannot entirely reverse these conditions.

Now, what we're talking about in this book is the small, minor imbalances that a general practitioner wouldn't be concerned about because they aren't severe enough to have a serious debilitating effect, but that certainly do have your body operating in sub-optimal conditions, and more importantly, the alkaline diet that can have it function far better than you ever imagined possible.

So in order to better understand how the alkaline diet will allow us to correct these small but important pH imbalances, we'll need to have a complete understanding of what could throw our pH out of balance and why it might happen.

As we have established a moment ago, the primary regulators of the body's pH level are the kidneys and the lungs. There are a large number of small systems in our bodies that have their own pH level and regulate them in their own ways, but the two main, body-wide regulators are the lungs and kidneys.

As you are likely already aware, we take in oxygen with our lungs when we inhale and expel carbon dioxide when we exhale. The oxygen that we take in is absorbed inside our lungs and used as fuel by our cells. The waste product that our cells produce by using the oxygen is carbon dioxide. Which is all very simple and pretty straightforward and familiar to all of us but here's the important part — carbon dioxide is slightly acidic. So by making slight adjustments to how much carbon dioxide is released or retained, our lungs are able to make adjustments to the overall acid-base level of our blood.

Similarly, the kidneys being the filtration system for the vascular system have the ability to excrete small amounts of acidic or basic compounds into the blood in order to make slight alterations to our blood chemistry. This is a slow process as compared to the more immediate effect of the lungs' pH regulatory system. So the lungs and the kidneys could be thought of as the short-term and long-term blood pH level regulators of our body.

If the blood pH level is out of balance, then it can lead to one of these two conditions — alkalosis and acidosis. With the standard balanced blood pH level being 7.40, anything below 7.35 is considered acidosis and anything above 7.45 is called alkalosis. Again, it is important to note that these are serious medical conditions and must be treated by a medical professional. It is always best to consult your doctor if you are suffering from these conditions. What we can do, however, is assist our body's natural pH regulation system by maintaining a blood pH level that is within the tolerable limits.

A low blood pH level or in other words, slightly acidic blood is far more common than the inverse and so that it is what we are primarily focusing on — an alkaline diet that will help us maintain a healthy blood pH level.

While any level measured at 7.35 and under is acidosis and needs professional medical treatment, it is far too common for our blood pH level to fall into that 'safe' range of 7.36-7.39 without being at that ideal sweet spot of 7.40. If you want to get the most out of your body, if you want your body to be operating at peak performance, and if you want to live your absolute healthiest life, then the 'safe' level of 7.36 is not tolerable for your body.

If you are truly serious about your health and your wellbeing, then the 'safe' blood pH level of 7.39 isn't even good enough for you. You need to have the absolute optimal blood pH level and you will settle for nothing but a perfect 7.40. Continue on reading in the next chapters and we are going to show you how.

Chapter 4: Why Alkaline is Best

If our body's pH level is all about balance, then why would maintaining an alkaline diet be superior to an acidic one? Shouldn't we be consuming a perfect balance of alkaline and acidic foods and nutrition? If those are among the questions you are now asking yourself, then you are on the right track. Those are great questions to ask.

There are several reasons why an alkaline diet is a crucial component in maintaining a healthy body and blood pH level. Remember that magic number? The ideal pH level for our blood that will allow our body to operate optimally? That is right — it was 7.40. And do you remember what the pH value for perfectly pure, unadulterated water is? That is right — it was a perfect seven. So what that means, of course, is that the ideal blood pH balance is in fact slightly alkaline at 0.4 units more basic than water.

So we can see already that in order to maintain our ideal pH balance, we will need to intake more alkaline foods than acidic foods. Of course, that is not to say that you can never consume anything acidic. In fact, it is important to have acids as well in order to maintain balance. We just need to be perfectly aware that our body does in fact require a slight alkaline balance and so we should be mindful of this when we plan our meals and overall diets.

This balance may also be reflected in the foods we choose to eat. They don't necessarily need to be extremely alkaline in order to transfer to us the health benefits we are looking for. They may only need to have a slight pull on the alkaline side of the scale. It all depends on our individual bodies and what they are in need of. And of course, everything scales. So a lot of a slightly alkaline substance may have the same value as a little of something with a higher alkaline value. Remember as well that the pH scale is logarithmic which is to say that each unit is exponential to the value of the previous unit. That means that consuming something with an alkaline value of nine would be ten times more alkaline than something with the alkaline value of eight. This is why we need to be careful when consuming anything that is alkaline or acidic. Things can become unhealthy or even dangerous in a real hurry. So, remember to plan ahead and do everything in moderation.

Another equally surface-level reason why it is important to consume a healthy amount of alkaline rich foods is because whether we are aware of it or not, many if not most of the foods we eat on a regular basis are either slightly or moderately acidic. Some very common foods and beverages even go as far as being highly acidic.

Now, again, it bears repeating that this does not mean that you cannot or should not consume these types of acidic foods and beverages at all. In fact, some of these acidic foods and beverages are very healthy and high in essential nutrients. The important thing, however, is to be aware of how much acidic substances we are consuming and how acidic those substances are.

Do you like fruit juices? How about coffee? Those are two great examples of highly acidic beverages that many of us consume on a regular basis. That is not necessarily a bad thing but just think about this — are you taking in the necessary amount of alkaline foods or liquids in order to maintain a healthy and optimal balance?

And what's more, it can often be a good deal more complicated than whether the particular food item that we are consuming is acidic or alkaline on a surface level. What makes the important difference is how the item we consume affects our blood pH level after it has been metabolized. And that could, in fact, be a good deal different than what it might seem to be based on the original acidity or alkalinity of the food item in question.

Another very important reason to remember to include alkaline foods in our diet in order to maintain a good acid-base blood balance is that an acid rich environment is considered by medical professionals to be a hotbed of disease and illness. And remember, it doesn't take much to become imbalanced in one's blood levels, so even a minor imbalance could quickly become a breeding ground for all manner of illness and health problems that you will absolutely want to avoid.

Just by remembering to consume a healthy and appropriate amount of alkaline foods and drinks, we can be safeguarding ourselves from any number of serious health concerns that could be lurking in our very blood. If you want to kill all of those potential illnesses dead before they become a real concern, you will need to act now and ensure that you are consuming an appropriate amount of alkaline foods.

This is the very topic that we will be going into next. We now know how important it is to maintain a good acid-base blood balance. We now know what that optimal blood pH balance is. And most importantly, we now know the dangers associated with having blood that is too acidic, and why it is so common for us to have a blood pH level that skews a little bit too acidic but not enough to go into full acidosis.

Equipped with this crucial information, we can now move on to learning about how to apply these factors to our everyday lives. Now, we are going to learn everything we need to know about how to create and maintain a balanced blood pH level, and all the tips and tricks to make it easy and straightforward.

Are you ready to have a body operating at optimal health? Are you ready to get the most out of your diet? Are you ready to prevent disease and illness that you didn't even know you were susceptible to?

Then continue on reading on, because all of your questions are about to be answered.

Chapter 5: Creating an Acid-Alkaline Balance

In this chapter, we are going to take a look at some of the biggest and best ways to gain control of your acid-alkaline blood levels and ensure that you can maintain them at an optimal level. Many of the things that we are going to talk about here are not just about diet. In fact, even the alkaline diet is not just about diet — it is about habits. It is about keeping good habits, maintaining regular health goals, and being in tune with your own body.

There are plenty of signs and symptoms that you may notice in the event that your body is too acidic. It is very likely that you will be experiencing chronic fatigue if your body is too acidic. Even if it seems that though you have been sleeping enough, you may still feel this way. Other symptoms of overly acidic blood are pain, headaches, joint pain, and stiffness.

Generally, people with acidic blood express an overall feeling of sluggishness and lethargy — sometimes even depression. It is also associated with a sense of irritability and a dulling of the mental faculties.

Obviously, if you are experiencing any of these symptoms, it will be in your best interest to correct them to the best of your ability. There are lots of ways to make your blood more alkaline and we will look at a few here.

First of all, you will want to make sure that your symptoms or feelings are in fact coming from a pH imbalance. In order to do that, you will need to check your blood pH levels regularly in order to maintain an up-to-date record of your pH levels. You can do this very easily with simple, inexpensive home testing kits available online and at many drug stores. You can get an instant and highly accurate reading and find out exactly where your body's pH balance is sitting. These simple test kits can help you make healthy and informed decisions about your personal health based on accurate and current information. This is a great, convenient, and inexpensive way to always be on top of your health.

Now, before we get into specific diet plans, let us talk about some changes that we can make to our diet in a general sense that will help improve our blood pH levels. One such thing that we can do to ensure that we are maintaining appropriate levels of acidity in our blood is by making sure that we eat more greens and dark-colored vegetables in general. Greens are not always the most popular foods to eat despite their great reputation and association with good health. But there are ways to make greens and other veggies fun and exciting and taste great.

You could try new recipes and try new types of veggies that you have never tried before. If you already love veggies, try to make sure that you get a good amount on a regular basis, if not every day. Even if you have a particular proclivity for veggies, it's easy to leave them out on occasion. Try to avoid that tendency.

And if you don't like veggies, maybe it has something to do with a reduction in their appeal on account of processed foods and excessive artificial sugars. Simply by cutting these things out of our diets as much as possible can dramatically reduce cravings for said items and make good, nutrient-rich foods like dark, green veggies far more appealing.

Either way, try to experiment with new ways of getting your veggies and making them fun and enjoyable. Try keeping some prepared in advance so that you always have a quick and healthy snack.

Here is another quick tip for general health and well-being. Every morning, the first thing you do when you wake up should be to drink a great big glass of ice-cold water as fast as you can. Why? Well, it's quick and it's easy, it costs nothing, and it has all kinds of great health and wellness benefits both short-term and long-term. First of all, the most immediate benefit is that ice-cold blast of invigorating water will snap you wide awake quicker and more effectively than any caffeinated beverage.

What's more, there's nothing better than an icy surprise to jump-start your body and kick your metabolism into a high-gear first thing in the morning. And because our friend water is completely calorie-free, that basically amounts to an energy boost and metabolism enhancer for free, metabolically speaking.

And do you want to take this brilliant life hack one step further and bring it into our alkaline friendly lifestyle? Add just a touch of lemon to that morning burst of water, or better yet, all the water you drink and you will get all the previous benefits plus that boost to your body's alkalinity that you need to function at peak efficiency. This may seem counter-intuitive given that lemon is acidic, but remember, it is not always about the acid-alkaline balance of the compound itself. It is how our bodies metabolize that compound. And lemon, being a well-known metabolism booster, will give you that alkaline push you need.

Of course, sometimes it is about the actual acidity of the food we are eating. Specifically, it is about the amount of acidic foods we are eating. If you find that you are suffering from symptoms of acid reflux, kidney stones, low bone density, or anything else associated with high body acidity levels — that is almost certainly a strong indication that you should be strictly limiting your intake of acidic foods.

This goes of course for any of the obvious culprits like tomato sauce or spicy foods, but there are some less obvious foods that metabolize into an acidic by-product in our bodies that we should be cautious of as well. This includes many processed cakes and cereals, often grain such as rice, oats or pasta, and even certain nuts like peanuts or walnuts. The key here is to just always be aware of what we are consuming and keep everything in moderation.

Beverages as well should be kept in moderation especially coffee and alcohol since both of which are associated with many negative health effects when consumed in excess, far beyond body acid-alkaline balance.

Chapter 6: Alkaline Diet for Vegetarians

Don't let the title fool you, this isn't just for vegetarians. The alkaline diet is great for anyone and everyone. If you are already a vegetarian — great, you are already in a great spot to maintain an amazing alkaline diet. If you're not a vegetarian, that's okay too. Remember in the previous chapter when we said that it is not necessarily about how acidic the foods we eat are but the quantities? Well, that goes for meat. Most meats are extremely acid forming in our bodies.

That means that while they may not be acidic to the taste or even particularly acidic on a pH test, they metabolize in our bodies into an acidic by-product. So naturally, most alkaline diet meal plans are going to be either vegan or vegetarian, or just very light on the meat and dairy. That doesn't mean, of course, that you need to completely remove meat from your diet, but if you choose to continue eating meat, you will need to be highly aware of the quality and quantity of the meat you consume. Keep it moderate and make sure to maintain good health otherwise and you should be okay.

But speaking of acid-forming diets, what so bad about them? We have seen some of the symptoms of having a seriously acidic blood pH level, but what if we're just prone to eating a little bit on the acid-forming side? Well, simply by virtue of the fact that we live in a modern world with modern luxuries and modern conveniences, most of our diets have strayed away from a good, healthy acid-alkaline blood balance, and maybe some of us without even knowing it is may be living with a chronic condition that results from such a diet known as 'chronic low-grade metabolic acidosis'.

This is what happens when our diet leans to the slightly acidic side for an extended, if not an indefinite amount of time. And the reality is that unless we take active steps to counteract this condition, it is highly likely that we will all succumb to it eventually, if not already. That is just the nature of the world we live in and the habits and practices of the industries and populations of our societies.

So if you are suffering from a form of low-grade chronic metabolic acidosis, perhaps without even knowing it, what are the signs? For one thing, you may notice some weight gain. This is a result of inefficient metabolic function on account of long-term low-grade acidosis. You may also suffer from pronounced but unspecific aches and pains. These will often be in the joints or even the bones. This type of pain associated with low-grade acidosis is likely the result of an acid buildup in the joints and bones.

Acid reflux, predictably, is also a good sign of this prevalent condition. But that is not the only part of your digestive system that can be affected. Long-term, low-grade acidosis can also cause a number of other digestive issues like intestinal cramping, irritable bowel, and generally poor digestion.

A whole host of other issues could manifest if you are one of the high percentages of people who unknowingly live day to day with a chronic case of low-level metabolic acidosis. Chronic fatigue and a general feeling of tiredness and muscle weakness may result. As can a number of other issues like skin problems, bone loss, kidney stones, receding gums, and urinary tract problems. So if you find that you have three or more of the many possible symptoms, then at least eighty percent of your caloric intake should be from alkaline-forming foods. The remaining twenty percent can more or less be of your choosing, but you may find high protein food items to be helpful.

A nice, quick and easy way to boost your body's alkalinity is by drinking beverages that are alkalizing. Spring water is one such naturally occurring source of alkalizing water. Also, water with a dash of lemon juice just as mentioned earlier. Green tea or ginger root tea will also have a similarly alkalizing effect.

You'll want to make sure that you are focusing primarily on eating whole foods. So that means vegetables and fruits, as well as root crops like potatoes and turnips. Also nuts and seeds can be an excellent alkalizing source and also a very strong source of protein. Beans are generally a good choice as well, although lentils, in particular, are renowned for their excellent alkalize boost. And when consuming grains, just remember that it is always best to consume whole grains.

Whether you are pursuing an alkaline diet to target a specific issue, or if you just want to have the healthiest body you possibly can, you are going to want to eliminate as much processed and artificial foods as possible. In fact, that goes for everyone, no matter what. Processed and artificial foods are doing anybody any favors, but they will certainly cause your body's blood pH level to lean to the acidic side. Refined sugars and added sugars rank very high up on the list of these types of foods that should be avoided at all cost. And refined white flour isn't doing you any favors either. In fact, some say it can be just as bad as refined sugars.

And while we are on the topic of eliminating things, if you can handle giving up coffee or any other caffeinated beverages, you will be giving yourself a major advantage on the path to a balanced blood pH level.

There are certain foods and nutritional elements that are acid-forming but that our bodies still need to function properly. These are things that we will have to keep a particularly close eye on in order to monitor amounts of intake. This includes essential fats, as well as pasta and other grains. If you are choosing to continue eating meat, then it should also be noted that meat and fish should both be consumed very sparingly and should also be very closely monitored and limited.

Finally, when it comes to dressing up your greens, namely when being consumed as a salad or being cooked, make sure to use high-grade and healthy fats like extra-virgin, cold-pressed olive oil, avocado oil, and coconut oil. All of which bring along tons of health boosts and benefits in addition to their alkaline-forming properties.

Chapter 7: Alkaline Meal Ideas

Now that we are fully informed and equipped to make good nutrition choices in regards to acid-alkaline blood balance, it is now time to put together some meal plans so we can put all of what we have learned into practice. We are going to look at a prime example of everything you might eat in a day to get the most out of your body.

This particular example isn't about limiting calories of eliminating any particular foods or food groups, so if you have any particular calorie counts you need to stay within, or if you are eliminating certain food groups from your diet such as meat or dairy, you may have to adjust accordingly. Just make sure that if you're replacing anything, to replace it with something of a similar acid-alkaline value, and that it serves that same food role as the replaced item. That is to say, replace proteins with proteins, carbs with carbs, et cetera.

And if you are not calorie counting, obviously use your best judgment here but there is no limit to how many alkalizing foods in the fruits and vegetable categories you can eat. Certainly, you should be limiting acidic foods like meats, dairies, grains, and processed foods if for no reason than to keep your acidity levels down, but fruits and vegetables especially the ones that are particularly alkalizing, you can eat to your heart's content.

So with that said, let's take a look at what our alkaline diet morning might look like.

We wake up nice and early in the morning, refreshed and ready to tackle our day because our healthy, alkaline-rich diet is allowing us to get the sleep we need and preventing our bodies from feeling overly fatigued. The first thing we do is get an ice-cold glass of water, squeeze some fresh lemon juice into it and drink the whole thing as fast as we can. As fast as we can without getting a brain freeze that is!

So now we're going to want to have a nice satisfying breakfast. Today, we are going to do a veggie scramble. Sounds great, doesn't it? This breakfast is going to consist of one or two eggs that we are going to scramble up with green onions, spinach or bok choy or any other leafy greens, and then some chopped bell peppers and diced tomatoes. You can even try it as an omelet if you like. Or even an egg-white omelet if you're feeling really healthy.

Or better yet, if you really want to go healthy, why not try that same breakfast, but as a tofu scramble instead of scrambled eggs. It's easy and delicious. Just replace the eggs with a handful of diced, firm tofu. You can season your tofu however you like, but we recommend trying a chili-style seasoning for some nice, tex-mex style breakfast burritos. Wrap optional.

After that amazing breakfast, we're going to have a nice productive and active morning. If we feel the need for a snack before lunch, we'll have maybe a fruit like an apple or a pear, maybe a banana or a handful of nuts or seeds. An ideal choice would be pumpkin seeds or almonds.

If you're anything like us, that already sounds like an amazing and healthy, nutritious day, but we haven't even gotten to lunch yet. So what might we enjoy for our midday meal on this ideal alkaline diet day? Why limit ourselves, let's look at a couple of options.

For one, we could try some lentil soup. This packs a nice alkalizing punch as it is but combine that with some steamed green like broccoli, carrots, onions, or kale, and you've got a powerful meal. Heck, why not steam up a mix of all of those veggies. Try a light olive oil-based salad dressing on the steamed veggies for some extra flavor.

As delicious as that sounds though, we still have another option. If you're still of the animal eating persuasion, you could try a nice big salmon steak, still a far healthier choice that its terrestrial cousin, served with some mixed greens which could include cucumber, carrots, tomatoes, and broccoli, among pretty much any other fresh veggies you would like. Similarly, you can season that with a light vinaigrette of your choice, but we particularly recommend a lemon and dill based one.

After all that amazing nutrition, you must be ready for a snack! Fight off that mid-afternoon slump with a nice alkalizing snack. This one you can keep nice and simple. Try a simple hard-boiled egg, seasoned with sea salt and fresh ground pepper to taste and a garnish of your choice if you're feeling fancy. Or if you're not inclined toward the animal-based foods, try a straightforward but delicious snack consisting of strips of sweet bell peppers, celery, or carrots, or a mix of all is always an option!

Finally, it's time for dinner and this is where you remaining meat eaters are going to have your way. You can have up to four ounces of your favorite meat, whatever that might be, but we highly recommend that if you must have meat, try to stick to something along the lines of fish, chicken, or other types of light poultry. You can serve this with a side of yam or sweet potatoes, baked or prepared in your favorite way and a nice simple garden salad with mixed greens and a light dressing of your choice.

Or for the plant-based folks, you can indulge in some pasta, but try to find or make pasta made from rice or quinoa, or other grains than wheat. Then you can top your pasta with all kinds of delicious veggies like broccoli, zucchini, and garlic. And then garnish with some olive oil and salt and pepper. Now you've had yourself a fresh and healthy food day!

PART IV

For all the meat lovers out there, the next diet that we are going to discuss is known as the carnivore diet.

Chapter 1: What Is Carnivore Diet?

The Carnivore Diet is the all-new trendy diet that expects its followers to go on a meat-only way of lifestyle. This diet completely goes against nutritional stereotyping. If someone asked you to replace that bowl of meat with vegetable oils and carbs, you probably have been misled!

This diet has won favor for several reasons and is, of course, not a fluke. If you find it attractive to sink in a carnivore way of eating, you have come to the right place.

The carnivore diet is the one that entirely revolves around a meat-based pattern of eating. It is one extreme diet that restricts you from eating plant-based foods and strictly opposes carbohydrate consumption. It might sound crazy, but there are people including Shawn Baker (the creator of this diet) who have normalized this fact that carbohydrate is a non-essential macronutrient, and there is no harm in cutting them down from the menu.

It is a zero-carb diet that altogether emphasizes consuming meat. Scientists consider this diet the best nutrition source for human beings, cutting out the chatter from plant toxins.

There are more anecdotes and testimonials than research backed up with science. This no-carb diet has also been a second option to those who have either failed to carry on with Paleo and Keto diet or have faced other severe consequences after following them. This is a bold claim and has a lot to unpack. Let's dive deep into the depth of its science.

Researchers have carried out several studies throughout the Earth that has proved its benefits on humankind.

- **Removes the Inflammatory Vegetables -** If you have been suffering from an autoimmune disorder or a damaged gut, this might be of concern.

  Almost every vegetable has some kind of toxin in it. Brussels Sprouts, broccoli, cauliflower have sulforaphane that causes hypothyroidism and damage to health. Nightshades damage carb and fat metabolism. Polyphenols cause DNA damage. Lectins cause leaky guts. Reservatrol can inhibit androgen precursors. Spinach has oxalates that may result in kidney stones, and the list goes on. Choosing a carnivore diet can be a game-changing plan for such people and others who are still being manipulated by conventional nutritional advice.

- **It Increases Cholesterol –** You all must have heard about bad and good cholesterol. Cholesterol plays a negative role when it is oxidized or damaged and gets trapped in the artery walls. LDL cholesterol, even though it is given the tag of the 'bad' cholesterol, protects your body from diseases and does not cause them. They bind to the pathogens allowing the immune system to expel them.

During inflammation, the body uses LDL as a protective mechanism. So, people with heart diseases have high LDL levels because it binds to the pathogens, getting rid of the damage ensuring that it does not spread. It is, in fact, the inflammation that causes heart diseases.

- **It Increases the Nutrient Density** - Animal-based foods have the most bioavailable form of nutrients that play a crucial role from growth to brain function. While you have been a fiber-freak, you might just have missed out on the essential nutrients. Vegetarians have a deficiency in Vitamin B12 and Iron. Americans have Vitamin D deficiency, and women have Calcium deficiency, while Zinc is a deficient nutrient worldwide.

The brain requires micronutrients, and it is animals that mostly provide this. Zinc and iron are vital nutrients that help brain growth, dopamine transport, and serotonin synthesis.

- **It Reverses Insulin Resistance -** The best thing you could do to your health is reverse the insulin resistance. It is a problem where your body's cells become unresponsive to insulin action and therefore refuse to stuff the cells with more energy, leading to a rise in insulin level. It occurs due to excess carbohydrates and fat that shut off the process of burning fat, causing the fat to be stored without being used directly. The carnivore diet can be a solution to this!

- **Weight loss -** Since protein-based foods are satiating, they allow you to stay distracted from eating by making you feel fuller. By ingesting protein, the primary energy source is shifted from carbohydrate to fat. It is similar to ketosis (adapted to fat consumption), where you can use your body fat instead of carbohydrate.

How to Start the Diet?

Although it is as simple as a diet can be, the initial weeks can be hard. Here are the things that you can incorporate to get through the changeover conveniently:

- Before starting with the diet, you can get your blood test done since the metabolic needs vary with every individual.

- You might feel like giving up at some point, start getting headaches, and experience fatigue. It is normal as your body will be getting used to using energy from fat rather than carbohydrates.

- Your eating desire might fluctuate. You will get adjusted to this form of eating after one week.

Chapter 2: Recipes for Tasty Appetizers

If you are a meat lover and want to start the carnivore diet, here are some recipes for you to follow.

Oven-Baked Chicken Wings

Total Prep & Cooking Time: 1 hour 5 minutes

Yields: 8 servings

Nutrition Facts: Calories: 348 | Carbs: 1g | Protein: 25g | Fat: 27g | Fiber: 1g

Ingredients:

- Half cup of grated Parmesan
- Four pounds of chicken wings
- One tsp. of salt
- One tbsp. of parsley
- A quarter cup of grass-fed butter
- Half tsp. of black pepper (ground)

Method:

1. First of all, the oven needs to be preheated to 180 degrees Celsius or 350 degrees Fahrenheit.

2. Take a parchment paper for lining the baking sheet.

3. Now, you need to take a shallow bowl or dish for melting the butter.

4. In another clean bowl, mix parsley, pepper, Parmesan cheese, and salt.

5. Once the herb and cheese mixture is ready, dip the chicken wings in the bowl of melted butter one by one. After dipping, roll the wings in the mixture.

6. Arrange all the wings properly on top of the baking sheet.

7. Bake for an hour.

8. Take out the baked chicken wings from the oven and serve them warm.

Steak Nuggets

Total Prep & Cooking Time: 55-60 minutes

Yields: 4 servings

Nutrition Facts: Calories: 350 | Carbs: 1g | Protein: 40g | Fat: 20g | Fiber: 2g

Ingredients:

- One pound of beefsteak or venison steak (cut it into chunks)
- Palm or lard oil (needed for frying)
- One large-sized egg

For Keto Breading,

- Half cup each of
  - Pork panko
  - Parmesan cheese (grated)
- Half tsp. of seasoned salt (homemade)

For Chipotle Ranch Dip,

- A quarter cup each of
  - Organic cultured cream (sour)
  - Mayonnaise
- More than one tsp. of chipotle paste (for taste)
- A quarter medium-sized lime (juiced)

Method:

1. For preparing the Chipotle Ranch Dip, you need to combine all the ingredients and mix properly. Use either more or less chipotle paste in accordance to your taste preference. Refrigerate the dip before serving for a minimum of thirty minutes. You may store the dip for nearly a week.

2. Take a large-sized bowl and combine parmesan cheese, seasoned salt, and pork panko. Set aside after mixing evenly.

3. Now, beat one egg. Place the breading mix in one bowl and beaten egg in another.

4. Dip the steak chunks first in egg and then in the breading mix. Then, place them on a plate or sheet pan lined with wax paper.

5. Before frying, freeze the raw breaded steak bites for half an hour. By doing so, the breading won't lift at the time of frying.

6. Heat the lard to 325 degrees Fahrenheit. Fry the chilled or frozen steak nuggets for nearly two to three minutes until you get the brown color.

7. Keep the fried nuggets on a plate lined with a paper towel. Sprinkle a pinch of salt. Serve hot along with Chipotle Ranch.

Grilled Shrimp

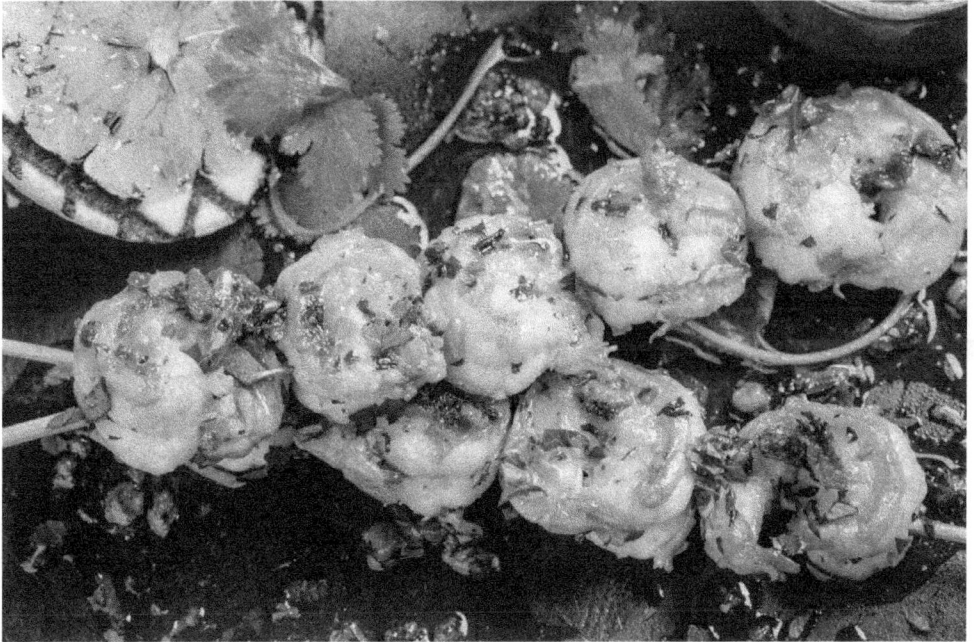

Total Prep & Cooking Time: 10 minutes

Yields: 4 servings

Nutrition Facts: Calories: 102 | Carbs: 1g | Protein: 28g | Fat: 3g | Fiber: 0g

Ingredients:

For grilling,

- One lb. of shrimp
- One tbsp. of lemon juice (freshly squeezed)

- Two tbsps. of olive oil (extra-virgin)
- For frying – vegetable oil or canola oil

For the shrimp seasoning,

- Half a tsp. of cayenne pepper
- One tsp. each of
  - Italian seasoning
  - Kosher salt
  - Garlic powder

Method:

1. You have to preheat your grill for this recipe on high.

2. Take a mixing bowl of large size, add all the ingredients of the seasoning in it and mix them well. Drizzle the lemon juice and olive oil into the mixture and keep stirring until you get a paste.

3. Add the shrimp into the bowl of seasonings and keep tossing so that all the pieces are evenly coated. Take the shrimp pieces and thread them onto wooden skewers.

4. Coat your grill with canola oil. You have to grill the shrimp for about three minutes for each side until they become opaque and pink.

5. Serve and enjoy!

Notes: You can store the grilled shrimp in the refrigerator for up to three days if you want to, but for the best flavor, you should consume it on the same day.

Roasted Bone Marrow

Total Prep & Cooking Time: 20 minutes

Yields: 2 servings

Nutrition Facts: Calories: 440 | Carbs: 0g | Protein: 4g | Fat: 48g | Fiber: 0g

Ingredients:

- To season – freshly ground black pepper and sea salt flakes
- Four bone marrow halves

Method:

1. Set the temperature of your oven to 350 degrees F and preheat.

2. Take a baking tray with deep sides and then place the bone marrow pieces in it.

3. Bake the bone marrow for half an hour until they become crispy and golden brown in color. The fat that is present in excess should have rendered off by now.

4. Season with black pepper and sea salt flakes.

5. You can spread the marrow separately on top of steaks, or you can serve the bone marrow as an appetizer.

Bacon-Wrapped Chicken Bites

Total Prep & Cooking Time: 30 minutes

Yields: 4 servings

Nutrition Facts: Calories: 230 | Carbs: 5g | Protein: 22g | Fat: 13g | Fiber: 1g

Ingredients:

- Three tbsps. of garlic powder
- Eight slices of thin bacon (slice them into one-third pieces)
- One chicken breast (large-sized, cut into bite-sized pieces)

Method:

1. Set the temperature of the oven to 400 degrees F and use aluminum foil to line the baking tray—Preheat the oven.

2. In a bowl, add the garlic powder. Take each chicken piece and dip it into the garlic powder.

3. Now, take each short piece of bacon and wrap it around the piece of chicken. Keep these prepared chicken pieces on the baking tray. Make sure they are not touching each other.

4. Bake the preparation for half an hour, and by the end of it, the bacon should turn crispy. After about fifteen minutes through pieces, turn the pieces over.

Salami Egg Muffins

Total Prep & Cooking Time: 25 minutes

Yields: 12 servings

Nutrition Facts: Calories: 142 | Carbs: 1g | Protein: 12g | Fat: 10g | Fiber: 0g

Ingredients:

- Four eggs (large-sized)
- Twenty slices of salami (uncured)
- Half a tsp. of kosher salt
- A quarter tsp. of black pepper
- Olive oil

Method:

1. Set the temperature of the oven to 350 degrees F and preheat. Take ramekins of four ounces each and spray them with olive oil. Then, place these ramekins on the baking sheet.

2. On the bottom of each ramekin, place one slice of salami and then on the sides, arrange four slices so that they are overlapping each other.

3. In this way, you will get a basket of salami, and in the middle of the basket, break one egg. Form four such baskets. Season the baskets with pepper and salt.

4. Bake the prepared salami baskets for twenty minutes, and by that time, they should be set.

5. Around the edges of the muffins, run a knife, and the muffins will get released. Serve and enjoy!

3-Ingredients Scotch Eggs

Total Prep & Cooking Time: 40 minutes

Yields: 12 servings

Nutrition Facts: Calories: 270 | Carbs: 1g | Protein: 19g | Fat: 20g | Fiber: 5g

Ingredients:

- Twelve large-sized boiled eggs
- Two pounds of chicken sausage or ground beef
- Two tsps. of salt

Method:

1. Preheating the oven to a temperature of 175 degrees Celsius or 350 degrees Fahrenheit is the first step for preparing such a delicious appetizer.

2. Line two baking sheets (small rimmed) with a parchment paper.

3. Take a large-sized bowl and combine chicken or beef and salt. Mix both the ingredients together by using your hands and then form twelve meatballs with it. Press the meatballs flat after placing them on top of the lined sheets.

4. Now, place each boiled egg inside each circle of flattened meat. After placing the eggs, start wrapping the meat nicely around the eggs. You are not supposed to leave any holes or gaps.

5. You need to bake for nearly fifteen minutes. Flip over as soon as the top looks cooked and again bake for ten minutes. If you want a crispy shell, then finish it under a broiler for approximately five minutes.

Notes: If you are willing to enhance the taste, then you may feel free to add any of your favorite herbs, such as garlic or rosemary powder. Add one tsp. of your preferred herb into the meat just before wrapping the eggs. Hard-boiled eggs are better in this case as it is difficult to peel the soft boiled eggs.

Chapter 3: Quick and Easy Everyday Recipes

Carnivore Waffles

Total Prep & Cooking Time: 6 minutes

Yields: 1 serving

Nutrition Facts: Calories: 274 | Carbs: 1g | Protein: 23.6g | Fat: 20.2g | Fiber: 0.8g

Ingredients:

- One-third cup of mozzarella cheese
- One egg
- Half cup of pork rinds (ground)
- A pinch of salt

Method:

1. For preparing the carnivore waffles, all you need is a waffle maker. First of all, preheat your waffle maker (medium-high heat).

2. Take a medium-sized bowl and whisk the pork rinds, cheese, and salt together.

3. Once you are done with the whisking part, pour the already prepared waffle mixture in the middle of the waffle maker's iron.

4. Close it and allow it to cook for three to five minutes. Or, you may cook until the waffle gets an attractive golden brown color.

5. Now, remove the cooked waffle and serve hot.

Notes: *The carnivore waffle will turn out to be more delicious if you place a cube of butter or runny egg on top of it. Greasing the waffle maker is not required before you start cooking waffles.*

Chicken Bacon Pancakes

Total Prep & Cooking Time: 20 minutes

Yields: 4 servings

Nutrition Facts: Calories: 444 | Carbs: 0g | Protein: 33g | Fat: 34g | Fiber: 0g

Ingredients:

- Four bacon slices
- Two chicken breasts
- Two tbsps. of coconut oil
- Four eggs (medium-sized, whisked)

Method:

1. First, you need to add all the ingredients to the bowl of the food processor except for the oil and then process everything together to form a smooth mixture.

2. After that, take your frying pan, and coconut oil to it.

3. From the batter that you just made, form four pancakes.

4. Fry these pancakes until they are set and properly cooked. Do the same with the rest of the batter.

Garlic Cilantro Salmon

Total Prep & Cooking Time: 25 minutes

Yields: 4 servings

Nutrition Facts: Calories: 294 | Carbs: 1g | Protein: 38.9g | Fat: 14.2g | Fiber: 0g

Ingredients:

- One lemon
- One fillet of salmon (large)
- A quarter cup of cilantro leaves (freshly chopped)
- Four garlic cloves (minced)
- One tablespoon of butter (optional)
- To taste – freshly ground black pepper and kosher salt

Method:

1. Set the temperature of the oven to 400 degrees F and preheat. Take a baking sheet and line it with foil. Place the fillets of salmon on it. You don't have to grease the foil.

2. Sprinkle the juice of one lemon over the fillet of salmon. Spread cilantro and garlic on top of the fillets evenly and season with pepper and salt. If you want to use butter, then you have to place thin slices on top of the salmon fillet at this stage.

3. Now, place the salmon along with the foil in the oven and bake for about seven minutes.

4. Set broil settings and cook the salmon for an additional seven minutes. The top part should become crispy.

5. Use a flat spatula to remove the salmon from the oven. Separate the skin from the fish and serve!

Mustard-Seared Bacon Burgers

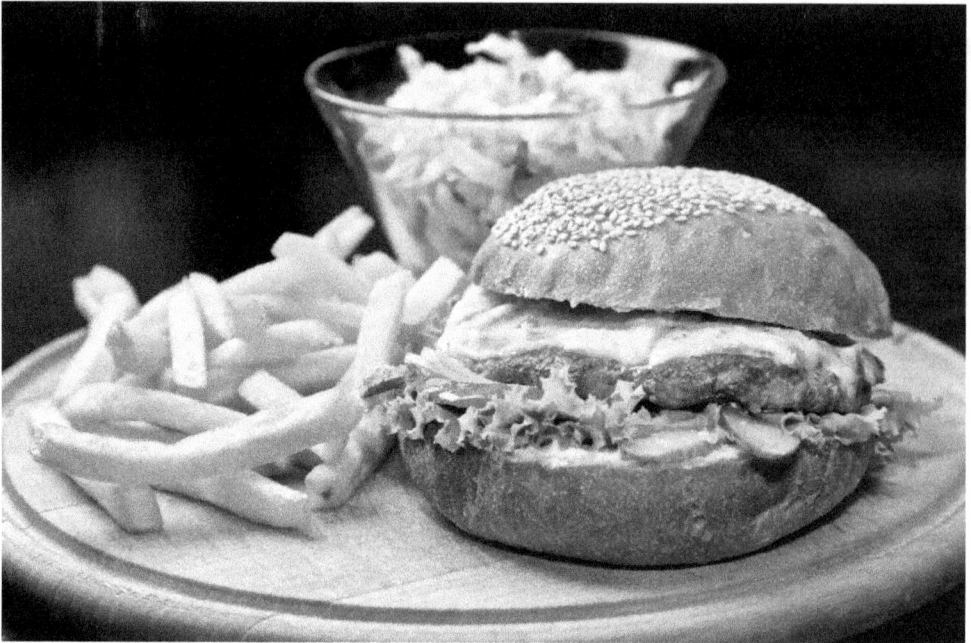

Total Prep & Cooking Time: 30 minutes

Yields: 6 servings

Nutrition Facts: Calories: 525 | Carbs: 3g | Protein: 22g | Fat: 45g | Fiber: 4g

Ingredients:

- 1.5 pounds of ground beef
- Four ounces of diced bacon
- Six tbsps. of yellow mustard
- To taste – salt and pepper

For the toppings,

- One tomato (properly diced)
- Half a red onion (diced)
- One avocado (thinly sliced)

For the sauce,

- Two tsps. of yellow mustard
- One tsp. of tomato paste
- A quarter cup of mayo

Method:

1. Take a pan and cook the bacon in it until it becomes crispy. You have to keep the grease of the bacon separately so that it can be used later. Then, take the bacon bits and keep them in a bowl along with the ground beef. Use pepper and salt to season them.

2. You will be able to form six patties from the mixture.

3. Now, you have to fry these burger patties on high flame so that they can get a great color. If you want, you can also choose to grill them.

4. Each patty will then have to be coated with one tbsp. of mustard and then, place the patty on the pan with the mustard-side facing down. Sear the patties one by one.

5. Take another bowl in which you can mix all the ingredients of the sauce together.

6. Each burger patty will have to be coated with sauce, and then, you can top them with slices of avocado, tomato, and onions.

Crockpot Shredded Chicken

Total Prep & Cooking Time: 6 hours

Yields: 8 servings

Nutrition Facts: Calories: 201 | Carbs: 1g | Protein: 24g | Fat: 10g | Fiber: 0g

Ingredients:

- Four garlic cloves
- Four chicken breasts
- One cup of chicken broth
- Half an onion (sliced)
- One tbsp. of Italian seasoning
- To taste – Salt and pepper

Method:

1. Take all the ingredients and add them to the crockpot.

2. Cook them for about six hours on low.

3. Use forks to shred the meat.

4. You can enjoy the shredded chicken with a variety of dishes like sautés, lettuce wraps, salads, or even soups.

Chapter 4: Weekend Dinner Recipes

Organ Meat Pie

Total Prep & Cooking Time: 20 minutes

Yields: 4 servings

Nutrition Facts: Calories: 412 | Carbs: 2g | Protein: 35g | Fat: 28g | Fiber: 4.2g

Ingredients:

- Half pound each of
  - Beef liver (ground)
  - Beef heart (ground)
  - Ground beef
- Three eggs
- Butter, ghee or Homemade Tallow or any melted cooking fat
- Salt (as required)

Method:

1. The oven needs to be preheated to 175 degrees Celsius or 350 degrees Fahrenheit.

2. Take a mixing bowl: mix ground beef, beef heart, and beef liver along with eggs and cooking fat of your choice. Lastly, add salt into the mixture.

3. Now, take a pie plate of nine inches and grease it lightly. Pour the mixture into the pie plate evenly.

4. Bake it for nearly fifteen to twenty minutes. Or, you may bake until the egg is totally set.

5. After baking, remove the pie from direct heat and let it cool for about five minutes. Serve it in a warm condition. In the case of leftovers, enjoy it cold.

Notes: *For those of you who are willing to add flavor to this recipe, you may add half tbsp. of any seasoning mix with the meat.*

Smokey Bacon Meatballs

Total Prep & Cooking Time: 30 minutes

Yields: 8 servings

Nutrition Facts: Calories: 280 | Carbs: 1g | Protein: 13g | Fat: 25g | Fiber: 0g

Ingredients:

- Two garlic cloves (skins peeled)
- Eight bacon slices (crumbled and cooked)
- One pound ground chicken or two chicken breasts
- One egg (properly whisked)
- Two drops of liquid smoke
- One tbsp. of onion powder
- Four tbsps. of olive oil

Method:

1. First, take all the ingredients (except for the oil) and add them to the bowl of the food processor and mix everything.

2. You will be able to form about twenty to twenty-four meatballs from the mixture. These balls will be small in size.

3. Now, take a large-sized frying pan, and then heat the oil. Add the meatballs and fry them until they are browned. It will take about five minutes for each side. If you want them to be perfect, then avoid overcrowding and cook in batches.

Steak au Poivre

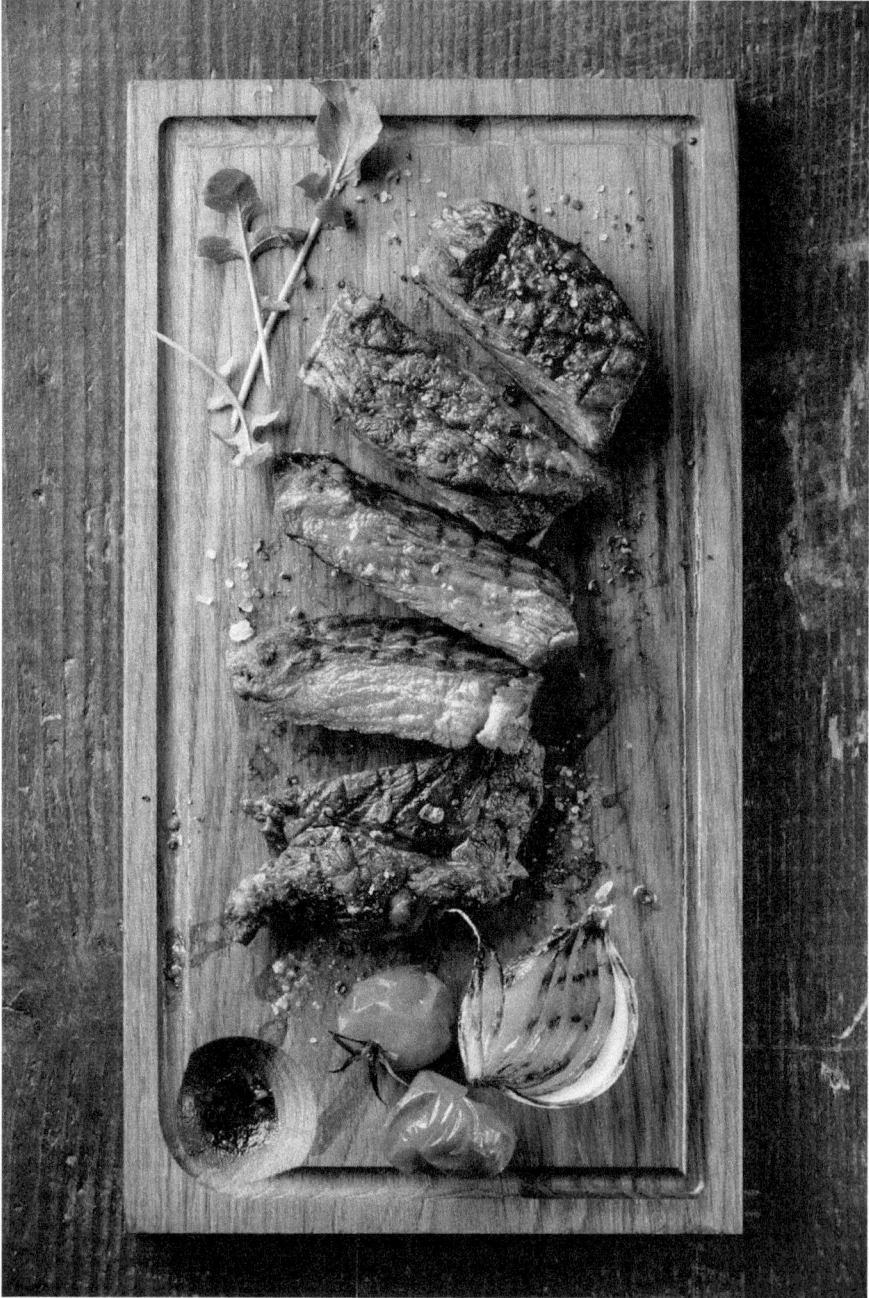

Total Prep & Cooking Time: 15 minutes

Yields: 1 serving

Nutrition Facts: Calories: 696 | Carbs: 2g | Protein: 42g | Fat: 58g | Fiber: 0g

Ingredients:

- One fillet of mignon (approximately six ounces)
- One thyme sprig
- One tbsp. of salt
- Two tbsps. each of
  - Ghee
  - Peppercorns
- Two garlic cloves (minced)

Method:

1. After you take the steaks out of the refrigerator, season them nicely with salt and then allow them to sit for about half an hour.

2. Use a mortar and pestle to crush the peppercorns completely on a pan or a flat board.

3. Take the steak, and on both sides of it, press the crushed peppercorns.

4. Place a skillet on the oven and heat it. Add the ghee. After that, sauté the thyme and garlic.

5. When you notice that the ghee has become hot, place the pieces of steak in the pan. Cook each side for about four minutes. The end result will be medium-rare steak.

Skillet Rib Eye Steaks

Total Prep & Cooking Time: 55 minutes

Yields: 2 servings

Nutrition Facts: Calories: 347 | Carbs: 1g | Protein: 22g | Fat: 14.2g | Fiber: 0g

Ingredients:

- Two tsps. of freshly chopped rosemary leaves
- One tsp. of seasoning of your choice
- One tbsp. each of
    - Olive oil
    - Unsalted butter
- One rib-eye steak (bone-in)

Method:

1. Take the sheet pan and on it, place the rib-eye steak. Use the seasoning to coat both sides properly. Spread the rosemary leaves on top.

2. Now, keep this steak in the refrigerator for three days after covering. Before cooking, take the steak out and keep it outside at room temperature for half an hour.

3. Place a skillet on the oven and heat it. Add olive oil and butter and wait until all of the butter has melted. Coat the skillet properly with butter by tilting the pan.

4. Now, add the steak to the skillet and cook for about five minutes until you notice that the bottom side has become caramelized and browned. After that, flip it over and baste the other side with oil and butter and cook it for five more minutes.

5. Take the steak off from the pan and slice it into thin pieces after it has cooled down for about five minutes.

Pan-Fried Pork Tenderloin

Total Prep & Cooking Time: 20 minutes

Yields: 2 servings

Nutrition Facts: Calories: 330 | Carbs: 0g | Protein: 47g | Fat: 15g | Fiber: 0g

Ingredients:

- One tbsp. of coconut oil
- To taste – pepper and salt
- One pound of pork tenderloin

Method:

1. Start by cutting the pork tenderloin in two halves.

2. Place your frying pan on the oven on medium flame. Add the oil in the pan and heat it.

3. Once the oil has melted completely, place the two pieces of the pork tenderloin in the oil.

4. Allow the pieces to cook thoroughly. Use tongs to flip the pieces so that all the sides of the pork are evenly cooked.

5. Take a reading on the thermometer, and it should show that the temperature is just below 63 degrees C or 145 degrees F.

6. Allow the pork to cool down after you take it out and then use a sharp knife to cut it into small pieces.

Carnivore Chicken Enchiladas

Total Prep & Cooking Time: 30 minutes

Yields: 10 servings

Nutrition Facts: Calories: 271 | Carbs: 5g | Protein: 25g | Fat: 7g | Fiber: 1.5g

Ingredients:

- Two chicken breasts (skinless, boneless)
- Three tbsps. of bottles lime juice + juice of one fresh lime
- One tsp. of dried garlic
- 16 oz. of sliced chicken
- Chimichurri sauce
- One jar of enchilada sauce
- One bell pepper (thinly sliced)
- Eight oz. each of
  - Cooked spinach
  - Shredded cheese

Method:

For making the shredded chicken,

1. First, take a crockpot and add the shredded pieces of chicken in it. Add the lime juice too.

2. Sprinkle the Chimichurri sauce on top of the chicken and then sprinkle the garlic on top.

3. Now, cook the chicken for about 4-5 hours if you want to cook it on high. Alternatively, if you're going to cook it on low, then set it for 8 hours.

4. Once it is done, use a fork to shred the chicken.

Assembling the enchiladas,

1. Set the temperature of your oven to 400 degrees F and preheat.

2. Take all the other ingredients like pepper and spinach and prep them.

3. The enchilada wrapped will be made by the four slices of chicken.

4. In the middle of the wrapper, add the shredded chicken.

5. Then, on either side, add the cooked spinach, pepper, and some of the cheese.

6. Roll the wrappers carefully and make sure they are firm.

7. Once you have rolled them completely, place them in a pan with the seam sides facing downwards. Then, add the enchilada sauce all over them.

8. Take the remaining portion of the cheese and sprinkle on top of the enchiladas. Bake the preparation for about fifteen minutes in the oven.

9. Serve and enjoy!

PART V

What Is Emotional Eating?

Emotional eating occurs when a person suffering from emotional deficiencies of some sort, including lack of affection, lack of connection, or other factors like stress, depression, anxiety, or even general negative feelings like sadness or anger, eats in order to gain comfort from the food they are eating.

Many people find comfort in food. When people experience negative feelings and turn to food consumption in order to reduce their pain or to feel better, this is called emotional eating.

Now, some people do this on occasion like after a breakup or after a bad fight, but when this occurs at least a few times a week, this is when it is considered to have a negative impact on one's life and is when it becomes an issue that needs to be addressed.

What Is Binge Eating?

Binge eating disorder is another disorder that can be seen along with emotional eating. Binge eating disorder is when a person eats much more than a regular amount of food in a single occasion or sitting, and they feel unable to control themselves or to stop themselves. This could also be defined as a compulsion to overeat. In order to be considered a disorder, it has to happen at least two times per week for longer than six months consecutively.

Along with binge eating is overeating, although this is also sometimes seen as a separate disorder altogether. Overeating is when a person eats more than they require in order to sustain life. This occurs when they consume much more than they need in a day, or in a single sitting.

Overeating does not necessarily become binge eating, but it certainly can. Overeating is a general term used to describe the eating disorders that we just defined-Emotional Eating and Binge Eating. Thus, overeating could involve binge eating, food addiction, or other food-related disorders. In this book, we will be focusing on emotional eating and binge eating, and how you can overcome these two food-related disorders.

What Is Bulimia?

Bulimia is another eating disorder. Bulimia involves binge eating, followed by extreme feelings of shame, guilt, and disdain for oneself and one's body. This is accompanied by intense feelings of body dysmorphia and body image issues, as well as the desire to be "skinnier." Thus, the person will turn to purging- or self-inflicted vomiting in an effort to lose weight and rid themselves of the guilt and shame.

Chapter 1: Understanding Your Food-Related Disorder

In this chapter, we are going to look at these two food-related disorders (binge eating/ bulimia and emotional eating) in much more detail. We will begin by looking at the most common reasons why people suffer from these disorders and will spend some time examining scientific research about why these disorders exist.

Why Do People Eat Emotionally?

The reason that emotional eating occurs is that eating foods that we enjoy makes us feel rewarded on an emotional and physiological level within our brain.

Why Do People Binge Eat?

People binge eat for a very similar reason to the reason why people experience emotional eating. This is because eating foods that we enjoy in terms of taste, smell, texture, and so on, makes us feel rewarded on an emotional and physiological level within our brains.

Throughout the rest of this chapter, we will look more in-depth at these eating disorders in order to give you more information about why they occur and what could cause them.

Scientific Research on Eating Disorders and Why They Exist

You may be asking how food cravings can result from emotional deficiencies and how these two seemingly unrelated things can be considered related. While we have touched on this briefly in this book already, the reason for this is that your body learns, over time, that eating certain foods makes it feel rewarding, positive, and happy for some time after it is ingested. These foods include convenience foods such as those containing processed sugars or salts, fast food, and quick pastries.

When you are sad or worried, your body feels negative and looks for ways to remedy this. Your brain then connects these two facts- that the body does not feel positive and that it wants to find a way to fix this. The brain then decides that eating the foods that make it feel good will remedy the situation. This process happens in the background of your mind without you being aware of it, and it leads you to consciously feel a craving for those specific foods such as sugary snacks or salty fast-food meals. You may not even be aware of why. If you then decide to give in to this craving and eat something like a microwave pizza snack, your body will feel rewarded and happy for a brief period of time. This reinforces to your brain that turning to food in an effort to make yourself feel better emotionally has been successful.

If you end up feeling down and guilty that you ate something that was unhealthy or that you ate too much, your brain will again try and remedy these negative emotions by craving food. This is how a cycle of emotional eating or a cycle of bingeing and purging can begin and continue. This could happen largely in your

143

subconscious without you being any the wiser.

Why Do People Have Bulimia or Other Food Disorders?

Because scientists and psychiatrists understand this process that occurs in the brain, they know that food cravings can indicate emotional deficiencies. While there are other types of cravings that can occur, such as those that pregnant ladies experience, or those that indicate nutrient deficiencies, there are ways to tell that a craving is caused by some type of emotional deficiency.

It begins by determining the foods that a person craves and when they crave them. If every time someone has a stressful situation, they feel like eating a pizza, or if a person who is depressed tends to eat a lot of chocolate, this could indicate emotional eating. As you know by now, emotional eating and bulimia are closely related, and emotional eating can lead to bulimia over time.

If you crave fruit like a watermelon on a hot day, you are likely just dehydrated, and your body is trying to get water from a water-filled fruit that it knows will make it more hydrated. Examining situations like this has led scientists and psychiatrists to explore eating disorders in more depth and determine what types of emotional deficiencies can manifest themselves through food cravings or disordered eating in this way.

In the next chapter, we will look at psychological triggers that can lead to disordered eating.

The Neuroscience of Brain Chemicals and Food As a Reward

Many times, we may see ingredients on the packages of foods we eat, but we aren't really sure of exactly what they are, just that they taste good. In this section, we will take a deeper look at them and what they do to your brain.

Casein is a heavily processed ingredient that is derived from milk. It is processed a few times over and eventually creates milk solids that are concentrated. These milk solids- called Casein are then added into foods like cheese, french fries, milkshakes, and other fast and convenient packaged or fast-foods that contain dairy or dairy products (such as pastries and salad dressings). Casein has been compared to nicotine in its addictive properties. It is often seen in cheese, and this is why there is increasing evidence that people can become, and many are already addicted to cheese. The reason for this is during digestion. When cheese and other foods that contain casein are digested, it is broken down, and one of the compounds that it breaks down into is a compound that is strikingly similar to opioids- the highly addictive substance that is in pain killers.

High fructose corn syrup is surely an ingredient you have heard of before or at least one that you have seen on the packaging of your favorite snacks or quick foods. While this is actually derived from real corn, after it is finished being processed, there is nothing corn-like about it. High fructose corn syrup is essentially the same thing as refined sugar when all is said and done. It is used as a sweetener in foods like soda, cereal, and other sweet and quick foods. The reason why this ingredient is seen so often is that it is much cheaper than using sugar and is much easier to work with. High Fructose Corn Syrup is another common food additive that has been shown to be highly addictive. This substance has been shown to be similar to cocaine in its addictive properties.

MSG stands for Monosodium Glutamate, which sounds a lot like a chemical you may have encountered in science class in college. MSG is added to foods to give it a delicious flavor. It is essentially a very concentrated form of salt. What this does in foods such as fast-food, packaged convenience foods, and buffet-style food is that it gives it that wonderfully salty and fatty flavor that makes us keep coming back for more. Companies put this in food because it comes at an extremely low cost, and the flavor it brings covers up the artificial flavors of all of the other cheap ingredients that are used to make these foods. MSG has been known to block our natural appetite suppressant, which normally kicks in when we have had enough to eat. For this reason, when we are eating foods containing MSG, we do not recognize when we are satiated, and we continue to eat until we are stuffed because it tastes so great.

Chapter 2: Understanding Your Mind

In this chapter, we are going to look at some of the psychological factors that can lead to disordered eating so that you can gain a better understanding of what could have led you to use food as a means of coping.

Psychological and Emotional Triggers

There are several types of emotional deficiencies that can be indicated by disordered eating. We will explore these in detail below in hopes that you will recognize some of the reasons why you may be struggling with an eating disorder.

Childhood Causes

The first example of an emotional deficiency that we will examine is more of an umbrella for various emotional deficiencies. This umbrella term is Childhood Causes. If you think back on your childhood, think about how your relationship with food was cultivated. Maybe you were taught that when you behaved, you received food as a reward. Maybe when you were feeling down, you were given food to cheer you up. Maybe you turned to food when you were experiencing negative things in your childhood. Any of these could cause someone to suffer from emotional eating in their adulthood, as it had become something learned. This type is quite difficult to break as it has likely been a habit for many, many years, but it is possible. When we are children, we learn habits and make associations without knowing it that we often carry into our later lives. While this is no fault of yours, recognizing it as a potential issue is important to make changes.

Covering Up Emotions

Another emotional deficiency that can manifest itself in emotional eating and food cravings is actually the effort to cover up our emotions. Sometimes we would rather distract ourselves and cover up our emotions than to feel them or to face them head-on. In this case, our brain may make us feel hungry in an effort to distract us from the act of eating food. When we have a quiet minute where these feelings or thoughts would pop into our minds, we can cover them up by deciding to prepare food and eat and convince ourselves that we are "too busy" to acknowledge our feelings because we have to deal with our hunger. The fact that it is hunger that arises in this scenario makes it very difficult to ignore and very easy to deem as a necessary distraction since, after all, we do need to eat in order to survive. This can be a problem though, if we are not in need of nourishment, and we are telling ourselves that this is the reason why we cannot deal with our demons or our emotions. If there is something that you think you may be avoiding dealing with or thinking about or if you tend to be very uncomfortable with feelings of unrest, you may be experiencing this type of emotional eating.

Feeling Empty or Bored

When we feel bored, we often decide to eat or decide that we are hungry. This occupies our mind and our time and makes us feel less bored and even feel positive and happy. We also may eat when we are feeling empty. When we feel empty the food will quite literally be ingested in an effort to fill a void, but as we know, the food will not fill a void that is emotional in sort, and this will lead to an unhealthy cycle of trying to fill ourselves emotionally with something that will never actually work. This will lead us to become disappointed every time and continue trying to fill this void with material things like food or purchases. This can also be a general feeling of dissatisfaction with life and feelings of lacking something in your life. Looking deeper into this the next time you feel those cravings will be difficult but will help you greatly in the long term as you will then be able to identify the source of your feelings of emptiness and begin to fill these voids in ways that will be much more effective.

Affection Deficiency

Another emotional deficiency that could manifest itself as food cravings is an affection deficiency. This type of deficiency can be feelings of loneliness, feelings of a lack of love, or feelings of being undesired. If a person has been without an intimate relationship or has recently gone through a breakup, or if a person has not experienced physical intimacy in quite some time, they may be experiencing an affection deficiency. This type of emotional deficiency will often manifest itself in food cravings as we will try to gain feelings of comfort and positivity from the good tasting, drug-like (as we talked about in chapter one) foods they crave.

Low Self-Esteem

Another emotional deficiency that may be indicated by food cravings is a low level of self-esteem. Low self-esteem can cause people to feel down, unlovable, inadequate, and overall negative and sad. This can make a person feel like eating foods they enjoy will make them feel better, even if only for a few moments. Low self-esteem is an emotional deficiency that is difficult to deal with as it affects every area of a person's life, such as their love life, their social life, their career life, and so on. Sometimes people have reported feeling like food was something that was always there for them, and that never left them. While this is true, they will often be left feeling even emptier and lower about themselves after giving into cravings.

Mood

A general low mood can cause emotional eating. While the problem of emotional eating is something that is occurring multiple times per week and we all have general low moods or bad days, if this makes you crave food and especially food of an unhealthy sort, this could become emotional eating. If every time we feel down or are having a bad day, we want to eat food to make ourselves feel better; this is emotional eating. Some people will have a bad day and want a drink at the end of the day, and if this happens every once in a while, it is not necessarily a problem with emotional eating. The more often it happens, the more often it is emotional eating. Further, we do not have to give in to the cravings for it to be considered emotional eating. Experiencing the cravings often and in tandem with negative feelings in the first place is what constitutes emotional eating.

Depression

Suffering from depression also can lead to emotional eating. Depression is a constant low mood for a period of months on end, and this low mood can cause a person to turn to food for comfort and a lift in spirit. This can then become emotional eating in addition to and because of depression.

Anxiety

Having anxiety can lead to emotional eating, as well. There are several types of anxiety, and whether it is general anxiety (constant levels of anxiety), situational anxiety (triggered by a situation or scenario), it can lead to emotional eating. You have likely heard of the term *comfort food* to describe certain foods and dishes. The reason for this is because they are usually foods rich in carbohydrates, fats, and heavy in nature. These foods bring people a sense of comfort. These foods are often turned to when people suffering from anxiety are emotionally eating because these foods help to temporarily ease their anxiety and make them feel calmer and more at ease. This only lasts for a short period of time; however, before their anxiety usually gears up again.

Stress

Stress eating is probably the most common form of emotional eating. While this does not become an issue for everyone experiencing stress, and many people will do so every once in a while, it is a problem for those who consistently turn to food to ease their stress. Some people are always under stress, and they will constantly be looking for ways to ease their stress. Food is one of these ways that people use to make themselves feel better and to take their minds off of their stress. As with all of the other examples we have seen above, this is not a lasting resolution, and it becomes a cycle. Similar to the cycle diagram we saw above, the same can be used for stress except instead of a negative emotion and eating making you feel more down, stress eating can make you feel more stress as you feel like you have done something you shouldn't have which causes you stress, and the cycle ensues.

Recognizing your triggers is important because this will allow you to notice when you may be feeling emotional hunger and when you are feeling actual hunger. If you become hungry, you can look back on your day or on the last hour and determine if any of your triggers were present. If they were, then you will be able to determine that you are likely experiencing emotional hunger, and you can take the appropriate steps instead of giving in to the cravings blindly.

There are many different emotional causes for the cravings we experience. There may be others than those listed above, and these are all valid. A person's emotional eating experience is unique and personal and could be caused by any number of things. You may also experience a combination of emotional deficiencies listed above, or one of those listed above in addition to others. Many of these can overlap, such as anxiety and depression, which are often seen together in a single person. The level of these emotional deficiencies that you experience could indicate the level of emotional eating that you struggle with. Whatever your experience and your struggles though, there is hope of recovery, and this is what the rest of this book will focus on.

Chapter 3: How to Stop Binge Eating, Bulimia, and Emotional Eating

In this chapter, we are going to look at how you can begin to tackle your mind in order to make positive changes for your body and break free from your eating disorder once and for all.

Addressing the Core Wounds

The key to solving these food-related issues is to address your core wounds. Understanding how your mind works will help you to better take care of it. You will be able to recognize your feelings and how they could have come about, and then treat them in a way that will help it to feel better. Bettering your relationship with food and your body will also improve your relationship with your mind. This will then allow you to begin to feed it what it needs, which will, in turn, lead to better cognitive functioning, control over impulses, and decision-making. This will help overall in your relationship with your food, your body, and your mind.

What Are Core Wounds?

As we discussed in the previous chapter, there are several types of emotional deficiencies that can be indicated by disordered eating. Once you have determined which of these emotional deficiencies (or which combination of them) are present in your life, you can begin to look at them in a little more detail. By doing so, you will come upon your core wounds. A core wound is something that you believe to be true about yourself or your life, and it is something that likely came about as a result of a coping mechanism you developed to deal with childhood. For example, this could be something like; the feeling of not being enough, the belief that you are unlovable, or the belief that you are stupid.

How to Address Them

By understanding and addressing your core wounds, you will be able to change your behaviors because of the intricate relationship that exists between your thoughts, your emotions, and your behaviors. By addressing your thoughts and emotions, you will change your behaviors and thus, free yourself from disordered eating. You may be wondering how you can begin to address your core wounds, as it can be difficult to know where to begin.

The first step is learning how to control and change your thoughts, which in turn, leads to changes in your behavior. By taking control of your thoughts and your beliefs, they don't have the opportunity to manifest into unhealthy behaviors such as overeating, turning to food for comfort, or any other unhealthy coping mechanisms that you have developed over the course of your life.

Becoming aware of your own thoughts is the most crucial step in this entire guide, as everything else will fail without it. Paying attention to your thoughts will help you identify what thoughts are going through your mind during an intense emotional moment. By looking deep within, in order to get in touch with your deepest feelings, you will be more likely to succeed in your weight loss and your overall lifestyle improvement.

One great example of how to put this into practice is through the use of journaling. Journaling can help in a process such as this because it can help you to organize your thoughts and feelings and will help you to see visually what is working and what isn't working for you. While we can give tips and examples, every person is different, so to find exactly what works for you, you will have to try some different things and see which techniques help you personally the most and in the best way. Journaling can be about anything like how you feel since beginning a new program, how you feel physically since changing your diet, how you feel emotionally now that you are not reaching for food in order to comfort your emotions and anything along the lines of this.

Positive Self-Talk

Once you have addressed your emotions and your core wounds, you can begin to intervene and change them so that they result in healthier behaviors. You will do this using positive self-talk. Adopting helpful thought processes fosters better emotions overall, which leads to more productive behaviors.

When people have developed unhelpful thinking processes, it is hard to make decisions to benefit their future selves because their thoughts create negative emotions that drive away motivation. This is where something called *positive self-talk* can come in. Positive self-talk can be instrumental in helping you to recover from disordered eating.

What Is Positive Self-Talk?

Many people's minds are controlled by their inner critic. The inner critic shares words with you, such as "You should just give up" Or "What makes you think you'll succeed?" which is rooted in the opposite of positive self-talk- Negative self-talk!

Instead of creating an open space that allows for mistakes, growth, and development, your inner critic causes you to question your worth, which makes it difficult for you to have the positive, growth mindset that is needed to complete tasks and go after things that may be difficult to achieve. In this case, helping your mind to begin using positive self-talk will help you to recover for the long-term.

How to Use Positive Self-Talk?

Below are several ways that you can begin to use positive self-talk. Over time, your mind will get used to thinking in this way, and you will find it much easier to do.

1. Remind yourself

Bad habits are built through many years, and no amount of willpower can undo a lifetime of bad habits, such as a strong inner critic that uses negative self-talk. By rewiring your brain to minimize the amount of negativity you feel in the first place, you will eventually get used to filling your mind with positive thoughts instead of negative ones.

2. Stop the automatic process of negativity

Often times, if the person had just paid attention to their thought process, they would be able to catch themselves before their mind automatically spiraled to a place of complete de-motivation. By catching yourself before you get there, you can prevent yourself from falling into your negative thought patterns that are limiting you and holding you back.

3. Find positive influences

Surrounding yourself with people that can encourage you and foster positivity will also change your inner-critic's opinion. Often times, hearing positive compliments from other people hold a heavier weight in the eyes of your inner-critic compared to you telling your inner-critic the same thing. Try spending time with people who are supportive of your goals and the changes that you are looking to make in your life. It will make your journey a little bit easier.

4. Limit Negative Influences

By limiting the negative influences in your life, you are making a statement to yourself that you place importance on preserving your mental health. When you remove negative influences and limit your exposure to things or people that make you feel negative, you are prioritizing yourself, and this is a great way to practice self-care.

5. Practice a gratitude exercise

This is a great exercise to remind yourself of everything that you love and appreciate about yourself and your life. Take time to write down all of the things that you love about yourself and about your life. This will remind you of all of the positivity surrounding you and will serve to uplift you.

Chapter 4: Making Healthier Decisions Using Intuitive Eating

This chapter will provide you with a solid foundation of knowledge on which to build your new lifestyle. We will look at how intuitive eating can be the answer to all of your struggles and help you to find recovery.

Making Good Choices

As we discussed in the previous chapter, making good choices begins with self-exploration and a deep look into your core wounds. Once you have done this, you can begin to make decisions that are positive for your health and your life, and over time these will become more and more habitual. We are going to spend this chapter looking at some of the ways that you can begin to make good choices related to food and eating.

How to Begin Making Good Choices Using Intuitive Eating

One great way to make good choices when it comes to food is by using something called intuitive eating. Below, I will define intuitive eating for you and give you some insight into how this can change your life.

What Is Intuitive Eating?

Intuitive eating is a new perspective from which to view how you feed your body. This style of eating puts you in control, instead of following a list of pre-designed guidelines about when and what to eat. Intuitive eating instead encourages you to listen to your body and the signals it sends you about what, how much, and when to eat. This ensures that you are giving your body exactly what it needs when it needs it, instead of forcing it into a specific kind of diet.

Intuitive eating does not limit any specific foods and does not require you to stick to certain foods exclusively. Instead, it encourages you to learn as much as you can about what your body is telling you and follow its signals.

The two main components of the intuitive eating philosophy are the following; eat when you are hungry and stop eating when you are satiated. This may seem like a no-brainer, but in today's societies, we are very far from eating in an intuitive way, as odd as it may seem. With so many diet trends and numerous "rules" for how you should and should not eat, it can be difficult to put these ideas aside and let your body guide you exclusively.

Intuitive Eating and Hunger

Before we begin looking at the specifics of intuitive eating, we will look at the different types of hunger and how you can tell them apart. This will help you to distinguish when you are hungry and when you may be turning to food to soothe your emotional state.

Real hunger is when our body needs nutrients or energy and is letting us know that we should replenish our energy soon. This happens when it has been a few hours since our last meal when we wake up in the morning, or after a lot of strenuous activity like a long hike. Our body uses hunger to signal to us that it is in need of more energy and that if it doesn't get it soon, it will begin to use our stored energy as fuel. While there is nothing wrong with our body using its stored fuel, it can be used as a sign to us that we should eat shortly in order to replenish these stores. Perceived Hunger is when we think we are hungry, but our body doesn't actually require any more energy or for the stores to be replenished. This can happen for a number of reasons, including an emotional deficiency, a negative mental state, or the occurrence of a psychological trigger.

The philosophy behind intuitive eating is that if you wait until you are too hungry before eating, you will be much more likely to overeat or to binge eat. This is because, by this time, you be feeling ravenous instead of mildly hungry. If instead, you choose to adhere to your hunger and eat when your body tells you that it needs sustenance, you will be much more likely to eat just the right amount. As a result, your body will be satisfied rather than completely stuffed, and instead of feeling shameful and angry that you have eaten, you can feel happy that you have provided your body with what it needed. This requires you to listen to and respect what your body is telling you and then provide it with nutrients in order for it to keep working hard for you!

The Benefits of Intuitive Eating

One of the reasons that intuitive eating is such a successful and cherished form of eating is that it allows the body to lead the mind in the right direction when it comes to seeking out its needs. Below, we will look at the benefits of letting your body guide your eating choices.

- Allows the body to get what it needs

Did you know that your cravings could actually be giving you much more information than you give them credit for?

A craving is an intense longing for something (in this case food), that comes about intensely and feels urgent. In our case, that longing is for s a very specific type of food. When we have cravings for certain foods, it can actually mean more than what it seems.

While you may think that a craving is an indication of hunger or of a desire for the taste of a certain food, it may actually indicate that your body is low on certain vitamins or minerals. As a result, your body seeks out a certain food that it thinks will provide it with this vitamin or mineral. This reaches your consciousness in the form of an intense craving. In this case, the body is trying to help itself by telling you what to eat. For this reason, understanding your cravings could help you give your body exactly what it is longing for.

For example, if you are craving juice or pop or other sugary drinks like this, consider that you might actually be dehydrated and, therefore, thirsty. Sometimes we see drinks in our fridge, and since we are thirsty, we really want them. Next time you are craving a sugary drink, try having a glass of water first, then wait a few minutes and see if you are still craving that Coca-Cola. You may not want it anymore once your thirst is quenched.

If you are craving meat, you may feel like you want some fried chicken or a hot dog. This can indicate a deficit of iron or protein. The best sources of protein are chicken breast cooked in the oven, and iron is best received from spinach, oysters, or lentils. If you think you may not like these foods, there are many different ways to prepare them, and you can likely find a way that you like.

- Prevents overeating

It can be hard to know how much to eat and when you have had enough to eat without letting yourself eat too much. Sometimes people will eat until the point that they begin to feel completely full. Many times, we keep eating until we become stuffed, even to the point of making ourselves feel physically ill. Intuitive eating will help you to avoid this, as this kind of eating encourages you to give your body what it needs in order to take great care of it. Stuffing your body until it is too full is not what your body is asking for, and once you become accustomed to listening to your body's needs, you will know when it is time to stop.

- Helps you break free from self-judgment

intuitive eating will help you to finally make peace with your body and yourself as a whole. It does this by showing you that your body has needs and that there is no shame in tending to these needs, as long as you do so in a healthy way.

You cannot fully embrace and practice intuitive eating if you have those nagging feelings of self-judgment each time you take a bite of food or decide that you are going to eat lunch when you are hungry. For this reason, in order to practice intuitive eating, you must understand that feeding your body is an act of compassion for yourself and that this does not need to come with self-judgment.

- It is inclusive, not exclusive

One of the great things about this style of eating is that it is not founded on restricting a person's intake of certain foods or allowing only a small variety of foods.

Diets like this are extremely hard to transition to and are hard to maintain for a long period of time. Intuitive eating is about including as many natural whole foods as you wish, while also ensuring that you are consuming enough of all of your nutrients. With this style of eating, you can eat whatever you wish, whenever you wish. This makes it much easier to stick with this type of diet and reduces the chances of falling off after a short period of time due to cravings or intense hunger. It does not restrict calories or reduce your intake greatly, which makes it easier to handle than a traditional diet for many people. It feels natural to eat in this way, which makes it effective.

Chapter 5: Intuitive Eating Part 2

In this chapter, we are going to continue our examination of intuitive eating by looking at some more specific details related to this diet, as well as how to make it a regular part of your life.

How to Make Intuitive Eating Part of Your Life

One of the best ways to make this type of eating a part of your life is to practice it with intention. This is especially important when you are just beginning. Each time you feel a pang of hunger or a compulsion to eat, take a minute to examine your inner world. By doing this, you will get your mind and body accustomed to working together. In addition, do the same after you eat. By doing these two things, you will be able to ensure that you are eating when hungry and stopping when satisfied.

When you finish eating a meal, rank your level of fullness on a scale of 1 to 10, 1 being extremely hungry and 10 being extremely stuffed. This will help you to determine if you are successfully stopping when you are satisfied and not overeating.

It is also important that you learn how to deal with your emotions and feelings in an effective way without using food. Using the techniques that you have learned in this book, you will be able to address your inner demons, which will make space for you to listen to your body and its needs.

As you know by now, listening to your body, your emotions and your mind is extremely important when it comes to practicing intuitive eating. As long as you remember this, you will be well on your way to becoming a lifelong intuitive eater.

What Kind of Foods Should You Choose?

Fish is a great way to get healthy fats into your diet. Certain fish are very low in carbohydrates but high in good fats, making them perfect for a healthy diet. They also contain minerals and vitamins that will be good for your health. Salmon is a great fish to eat, as it is versatile and delicious. Many fish also include essential fatty acids that we can only get through our diet. Other fish that are good for you include:

- Sardines
- Mackerel
- Herring
- Trout
- Albacore Tuna

Meat and Poultry make up a large part of most Americans' diets. Meats and poultry that are fresh and not processed do not include any carbohydrates and contain high levels of protein. Eating lean meats helps to maintain your strength and muscle mass and gives you energy for hours. Grass-fed meats, in particular, are rich in antioxidants.

Eggs are another amazing, protein-filled food. Eggs help your body to feel satiated for longer and also keeps your blood sugar levels consistent, which is great for overall health. The whole egg is good for you, as the yolk is where the nutrients are. The cholesterol found within egg yolks also has been demonstrated to lower your risk of getting diseases like heart diseases, despite what most people think. Therefore, do not be afraid of the egg yolk!

Legumes are a great source of protein as well as fiber, and there are many different types to choose from. These include the following:

- All sorts of beans including black beans, green beans, and kidney beans
- Peas
- Lentils of all colors
- Chickpeas
- Peas

Examples of fruits that you can eat include the following:

- Citrus fruits such as oranges, grapefruits, lemons, and limes
- Melons of a variety of sorts
- Apples
- Bananas
- Berries including strawberries, blueberries, blackberries, raspberries and so on
- Grapes

Vegetables are a great source of energy and nutrients, and they include a wide range of naturally occurring vivid colors which should all be included in your diet.

- Carrots
- Broccoli and cauliflower

- Asparagus

- Kale

- All sorts of peppers including hot peppers, bell peppers

- Tomatoes

- Root vegetables (that are a good source of healthy, complete carbohydrates) such as potatoes, sweet potatoes, all types of squash, and beets.

Seeds are another great source of nutrients, vitamins, and minerals, and they are very versatile. These include the following:

- Sesame seeds

- Pumpkin seeds

- Sunflower seeds

- Hemp, flax and chia seeds are all especially good for your health

Nuts are a great way to get protein if you are choosing not to eat meat or if you are vegan. They also are packed with nutrients. Some examples are below.

- Almonds

- Brazil Nuts

- Cashews

- Macadamia nuts

- Pistachios

- Pecans

There are some **healthy fats** that are essential components of any person's diet, as the beneficial compounds that they contain cannot be made by our bodies; thus, we rely solely on or diet to get them. These compounds are Omega-3 Fatty

Acids, monounsaturated and polyunsaturated fats. Below are some healthy sources of these compounds:

- Avocados
- Healthy, plant-based oils including olive oil and canola oil
- Hemp, chia and flax seeds
- Walnuts

When it comes to carbohydrates, these should be consumed in the form of **whole grains**, as they are high in fiber, which will help to prevent overeating. Whole grains also include essential minerals- those that we can only get from our diet just like those essential compounds found in healthy fats. These essential minerals are selenium, magnesium, and copper. Sources of these whole grains include the following:

- Quinoa
- Rye, Barley, buckwheat
- Whole grain oats
- Brown rice
- Whole grain bread can be hard to find these days in the grocery store, as many brown breads disguise themselves as whole grain when, in fact, they are not. However, there are whole grain breads if you take the time to look at the ingredients list.

Nutrients You Need and How to Get Them

In this section, we are going to look at the most beneficial nutrients for your body and where/ how you can find them. This will help you to decide which foods to include in your diet so that you can ensure you are getting all of the nutrients that your body needs.

1. Omega-3 Fatty Acids

Some vitamins and nutrients are called "essential nutrients." Omega-3 Fatty Acids are an example of this type of nutrient. They are called essential nutrients because they cannot be made by our bodies; thus, they must be eaten in our diets. These fatty acids are a very specific type of fatty acid, and this type, in particular, is the most essential and the most beneficial for our brains and bodies.

They have numerous effects on the brain, including reducing inflammation (which reduces the risk of Alzheimer's) and maintaining and improving mood and cognitive function, including specifically memory. Omega-3's have these greatly beneficial effects because of the way that they act in the brain, which is what makes them so essential to our diets. Omega-3 Fatty Acids increase the production of new nerve cells in the brain by acting specifically on the nerve stem cells within the brain, causing new and healthy nerve cells to be generated.

Omega-3 fatty acids can be found in fish like salmon, sardines, black cod, and herring. It can also be taken as a pill-form supplement for those who do not eat fish or cannot eat enough of it. It can also be taken in the form of a fish oil supplement like krill oil.

Omega-3 is by far the most important nutrient that you need to ensure you are ingesting because of the numerous benefits that come from it, both in the brain and in the rest of the body. While supplements are often a last step when it comes to trying to include something in your diet, for Omega-3's, the benefits are too great to potentially miss by trying to receive all of it from your diet.

Magnesium

Magnesium is beneficial for your diet, as it also helps you to maintain strong bones and teeth. Magnesium and Calcium are most effective when ingested together, as Magnesium helps in the absorption of calcium. It also helps to reduce migraines and is great for calmness and relieving anxiety. Magnesium can be found in leafy green vegetables like kale and spinach, as well as fruits like bananas and raspberries, legumes like beans and chickpeas, vegetables like peas, cabbage, green beans, asparagus, and brussels sprouts, and fish like tuna and salmon.

Calcium

Calcium is beneficial for the healthy circulation of blood, and for maintaining strong bones and teeth. Calcium can come from dairy products like milk, yogurt, and cheese. It can also be found in leafy greens like kale and broccoli and sardines.

Chapter 6: How to Make These New Choices a Habit

Now that you have learned a wealth of information about intuitive eating, we are going to look at some strategies that you can use to make these new, healthy choices a habit. This will take time, but by employing these strategies, you will surely find success.

Healthy Thinking Patterns

In this section, we will look at a real-life example of dealing with challenges to demonstrate healthy thinking patters when it comes to intuitive eating.

Let's say you are trying to focus on healthy eating, and you find that you have had trouble doing so. Maybe you ate a cupcake, or maybe you had a soda at breakfast. From the perspective of traditional diet mentality, this would become a problem for the diet, and this would become a problem in your mind as well. You would likely be beating yourself up and feeling terrible about the choice you have made.

Let's look at this example in more detail. It is very important to avoid beating yourself up or self-judging for falling off the wagon. This may happen sometimes. What we need to do though, is to focus not on the fact that it has happened, but on how we are going to deal with and react to it. There are a variety of reactions that a person may have to this type of situation. We will examine the possible reactions and their pros and cons below:

- You may feel as though your progress is ruined and that you might as well begin again another time. This could lead you to go back to your old ways and keep you from trying again for quite some time. This could happen many times, over and over again, and each time you slip up, you decide that you might as well give up this time and try again, but each time it ends the same.

- You may fall off of your plan and tell yourself that this day is a write-off and that you will begin again the next day. The problem with this method is that continuing the rest of the day as you would have before you decided to make a change will make it so that the next day is like beginning all over again, and it will be very hard to begin again. You may be able to begin again the next day, and it could be fine, but you must be able to really motivate yourself if you are going to do this. Knowing that you have fallen off before makes it so that you may feel down on yourself and feel as though you can't do it, so beginning again the next day is very important.

- The third option, similar to the previous case, you may fall off, but instead of deciding that the day is a write-off, you tell yourself that the entire week is a write-off, and you then decide that you will pick it up again the next week. This will be even harder than starting again the next day as multiple days of eating whatever you like will make it very hard to go back to making the healthy choices again afterward.

- After eating something that you wish you hadn't (and that wasn't a healthy choice), you decide not to eat anything for the rest of the day so that you don't eat too many calories or too much sugar, and decide that the next day you will start over again. This is very difficult on the body as you are going to be quite hungry by the time the evening rolls around. Instead of forgiving yourself, you are punishing yourself, and it will make it very hard not to reach for chips late at night when you are starving and feeling down.

- The fifth and final option is what you should do in this situation.

This option is the best for success and will make it the most likely that you will succeed long-term. If you fall off at lunch, let's say, because you are tired and, in a rush, and you just grab something from a fast-food restaurant instead of going home for lunch or buying something at the grocery store to eat, this is how we will deal with it. Firstly, you will likely feel like you have failed and may feel quite down about having made an unhealthy choice. Now instead of starving for the rest of the day or eating only lettuce for dinner, you will put this slip up at lunch behind you, and you will continue your day as if it never happened. You will eat a healthy dinner as you planned, and you will continue on with the plan. You will not wait until tomorrow to begin again; you will continue as you would if you had made that healthy choice at lunch. The key to staying on track is being able to bounce back. The people who can bounce back mentally are the ones who will be most likely to succeed. You will need to maintain a positive mental state and look forward to the rest of the day and the rest of the week in just the same way as you did before you had a slip-up. One bad meal out of the entire week is not going to ruin all of your progress and recovering from emotional eating is largely a mental game. It is more mental than anything else, so we must not underestimate the role that our mindset plays in our success or failure.

By using this type of thinking, you will set yourself up for success and will not fall off of your plan completely after one slip up.

Healthy Lifestyle Changes

One important way to ensure that these healthy choices stick for good is by changing some aspects of your lifestyle. By doing this, you will reduce the chances of slipping up by eliminating them altogether. For example, you can change the way you approach the grocery store.

When you are entering the grocery store, it is important that you change a few things about the way you shop, in order to set yourself up for success. This is especially important when you are just beginning your intuitive eating practice, as it will be challenging for you to enter the grocery store and avoid cravings and temptations.

The first thing to keep in mind when grocery shopping for a new diet is to enter with a list. By doing this, you are giving yourself a guide to follow, which will prevent you from picking up things that you are craving or things that you feel like eating in that moment.

One of the biggest things to keep in mind when beginning a new eating practice like intuitive eating is to avoid shopping when you are hungry. This will make you reach for anything and everything that you see. By entering the grocery store when you are satiated or when you have just eaten, you will be able to stick to your list and avoid falling prey to temptations.

If you treat your grocery shopping experience like a treasure hunt, you will be able to cross things off of the list one at a time without venturing to the parts of the grocery store that will prove to be a challenge for you to resist. If you are making healthy eating choices, you will likely be spending most of your time at the perimeter of the grocery store. This is where the whole, plant-based foods are located. By doing this, and entering with a list, you will be able to avoid the middle aisles where the processed, high-sugar temptation foods are all kept.

Having a plan is key when it comes to succeeding in learning new habits and employing a new lifestyle. This plan can be as detailed as you wish, or it can simply come in the form of a general overview. I recommend you start with a more detailed plan in the beginning as you ease into things.

As everyone is different, you may be the type of person who likes lots of lists and plans, or you may be the type of person who doesn't, but for everyone, beginning with a plan and following it closely for the first little while is best. For example, this plan can include things like what you will focus on each week, what you will reduce your intake of, and what you will try to achieve in terms of the mental work involved.

Once you have come up with a general plan for your new lifestyle and how you want it to look, you can then begin laying out more specific plans.

Planning your individual meals will make it much easier for you when you get home from work or when you wake up tired in the morning and need to pack something for your lunch.

You can plan your meals out a week in advance, two weeks or even a month if you wish. You can post this up on your fridge, and each day you will know exactly what you are eating, with no thinking required. This way, there won't be a chance for you to consider ordering a pizza or heating up some chicken fingers because you will already know exactly what you are going to make. By approaching your new style of eating in this way, you can make this transition easier on yourself and ensure success every step of the way.

30-Day Meal Plan

The following 30-day meal plan includes a variety of meals that you can make in order to keep your first thirty days interesting and tasty!

Day 1

- Breakfast:

Coffee

Feta, mushroom and spinach, omelet.

- Lunch:

Oven-baked tempeh with broccoli and cauliflower rice.

- Dinner:

Chicken Caesar salad- tofu and romaine lettuce, parmesan

Day 2

- Breakfast:

Unsweetened yogurt with a mix of some berries such as strawberries, raspberries, and some seeds like flax seeds and chia seeds, and nuts like sliced almonds and walnuts.

- Lunch:

A healthy lunch-time salad with avocado, cheese, grape tomatoes, and a variety of nuts and seeds like spicy pumpkin seeds. Add a salad dressing on top such as blue cheese or ranch dressing, or a homemade one using olive oil and garlic.

- Dinner:

Chicken breast with onions and a homemade tomato sauce. Served alongside some grilled zucchini or eggplant.

Day 3

- Breakfast:

A no sugar added full fat Greek yogurt bowl with seeds, nuts and berries.

1 Cup of coffee

- Lunch:

Make your own lunch box, including firm tofu or meat of some sort, raw tomatoes, any type of cheese cubes that you wish, pickles, a hard-boiled egg, vegetables such as celery, carrots, radishes or zucchini, nuts for protein and fat such as walnuts, or almonds, homemade guacamole (avocado, onion, garlic, jalapeno).

- Dinner:

Grilled portobello, grilled eggplant and grilled zucchini as well as cherry tomatoes sautéed in extra virgin olive oil with garlic. Served with rice and protein such as pork or chicken.

Day 4

- Breakfast:

Coffee

Homemade mushroom & Spinach Frittata, including any vegetables that you wish such as bell peppers and onion.

- Lunch:

Cream cheese with cucumber slices for dipping.

Hard-boiled egg

Meatballs with sweet and sour sauce

- Dinner

Bacon, Avocado, Lettuce, Tomato panini.

Day 5

- Breakfast:

Egg Salad with lettuce, cucumber and whole grain bread.

- Lunch:

Homemade guacamole (avocado, onion, garlic, jalapeno, lime juice) with raw zucchini slices for dipping.

Hard-boiled egg

Tuna

- Dinner:

Cauliflower gratin (cheese, cauliflower, onion, garlic and so on)

As well as chopped lettuce drizzled with Caesar Dressing

Day 6

- Breakfast:

Coffee with heavy cream or coconut oil.

Celery sticks, dipped in peanut or Almond Butter

- Lunch:

Leftover cauliflower gratin

As well as chopped lettuce drizzled with Caesar Dressing

- Dinner:

Cooked or raw broccoli with grated cheese on top

Steak seared in olive oil

Day 7

- Breakfast:

Pancakes with fresh fruits

Black Coffee

- Lunch:

Cold pasta salad with fresh vegetables

Feta and Tomato Meatballs

Raw fresh spinach

- Dinner:

Spicy Spaghetti Squash Casserole

Fresh spinach, raw or cooked with 1 Tbsp ranch dressing drizzled on top.

Day 8

- Breakfast

Smoothie

- Lunch

Tempeh meatballs with guacamole and raw vegetable salad

- Dinner

Rice noodle stir fry with your choice of vegetables and tofu

Day 9

- Breakfast

Omelet cooked in coconut oil with cheese, onions, bell pepper and tomatoes

- Lunch

Tofu scramble with vegetables such as spinach and mushrooms and cheese

- Dinner

Curry with chicken, rice and coconut milk sauce with hot chili paste

Day 10

- Breakfast

Full fat yogurt unsweetened with berries, chia seeds, flax seeds

- Lunch

Cobb salad with boiled egg, vegetables of your choice, tofu, tempeh or chicken and Caesar dressing

- Dinner

Homemade pizza with your choice of toppings

Day 11

- Breakfast

Smoothie with chia seeds and flax seeds, berries and plant-based protein powder, as well as plant-based milk

- Lunch

Salad with tofu or boiled egg, olive oil dressing, spinach and diced vegetables

- Dinner

Vegetarian frittata using coconut oil, spinach, mushroom, cheese, bell peppers and tomato

Day 12

- Breakfast

Greek yogurt no sugar added with nuts and seeds

- Lunch

Homemade tacos with your choice of toppings, including ground turkey

- Dinner

Macaroni and cheese with crumbled roasted bread crumbs on top

Day 13

- Breakfast

Whole grain oats with no sugar added, nuts, flax and chia seeds as well as heavy cream and a plant-based nut butter.

- Lunch

Lettuce wraps with curried tofu and grilled eggplant and zucchini

- Dinner

Homemade burritos filled with crumbled, seasoned meat of your choice, sour cream, guacamole and diced tomatoes

Day 14

- Breakfast

Greek yogurt no sugar added with nuts and seeds

- Lunch

Avocado egg bowls with bacon

- Dinner

Fried rice with your choice of vegetables, scrambled egg and tofu

Day 15

- Breakfast

Coffee with heavy cream and no sugar added

- Lunch

Carrots with guacamole, cottage cheese with nuts and seeds and homemade baked zucchini chips with olive oil drizzle

- Dinner

Egg Salad with Lettuce Wraps

Day 16

- Breakfast

Pancakes with no sugar added maple syrup

- Lunch

Vegetarian egg quiche with spinach and mushroom

- Dinner

Broccoli salad with onion, a cheese of your choice, creamy ranch dressing, almonds and walnuts sliced, as well as some avocado and tofu cubes

Day 17

- Breakfast

Potato hash browns fried in olive oil, sunny side up egg and tempeh "bacon" with a side of grilled tomatoes

- Lunch

Avocadoes stuffed with cauliflower "taco meat", homemade salsa with tomatoes and herbs, sour cream, and grated cheese

- Dinner

Cooked or raw broccoli

Small amount of butter that can be added to the broccoli for taste

Grated cheese on top that can also be added to the broccoli

With steak seared in olive oil

Day 18

- Breakfast

Shakshuka with eggs, tomatoes and parsley

- Lunch

Grilled zucchini roll ups with tomato and cheese

- Dinner

Coconut milk curry with rice, bell peppers and tofu

Day 19

- Breakfast

Breakfast smoothie with berries, no sugar added and full fat milk

- Lunch

Broccoli and cheese fritters with homemade hummus to dip and a side of carrots, celery and cucumber for dipping

- Dinner

Cobb salad including hard-boiled egg, ham cubes, your choice of vegetables and an olive oil or ranch dressing

Day 20

- Breakfast

Spinach and mushroom frittata

- Lunch

Sandwich with scrambled eggs, spinach and mushrooms cooked in olive oil and topped with lettuce, tomato or any other fillings or toppings you wish to include. Finally, add a homemade creamy avocado sauce with avocado, cilantro, pepper and salt and some sour cream.

- Dinner

Rice risotto with cheese, vegetable broth and mushrooms

Day 21

- Breakfast

Unsweetened yogurt with a mix of berries such as strawberries, raspberries, and some seeds like flax seeds and chia seeds, and nuts like sliced almonds and walnuts.

- Lunch

Caesar salad- dressing with no sugar added

Raw vegetables, mixed greens and tempeh

- Dinner

Cauliflower gratin- cheese, cauliflower and choice of vegetables

Day 22

- Breakfast

Hash browns fried in olive oil, sunny side up egg and bacon with a side of grilled tomatoes

- Lunch

Stuffed half zucchini with feta cheese, tomato sauce (no sugar added) and herbs for topping

- Dinner

Mashed potatoes using whole milk and cheese, with grilled eggplant and mushrooms

Day 23

- Breakfast

Nut butter smoothie with yogurt, nut butter, flax seeds, chia seeds

- Lunch

Pan fried steak seasoned with herbs and olive oil, paired with

A spinach salad with raw vegetables of choice and no sugar added Caesar dressing

- Dinner

Cauliflower pasta salad with celery, spinach, onions, and walnuts

Day 24

- Breakfast

Feta, mushroom and Spinach, omelet

Coffee

- Lunch

Coleslaw with a creamy cilantro dressing, carrots, cabbage, celery, tomato and herbs for topping

- Dinner

Crispy tofu cubes with zucchini noodles and a homemade peanut sauce

Day 25

- Breakfast

No bake protein bars

Coffee with no sugar added

- Lunch

Roasted tomatoes with goat cheese, spinach, cilantro and olive oil & balsamic drizzle

- Dinner

Eggplant and zucchini "French fries" with olive oil and crispy tofu cubes

Baked chicken breast

Day 26

- Breakfast

Pancakes with no sugar added maple syrup, full fat Greek yogurt and berries for topping

- Lunch

Low carb broccoli cheese soup with crispy cauliflower on the side

- Dinner

Curried rice with choice of vegetables, such as bell peppers and broccoli

Day 27

- Breakfast

Breakfast salad with scrambled egg, avocado, mixed greens, grilled tomatoes and cheese

- Lunch

Fried goat cheese with roasted red peppers, spinach and olive oil drizzle

- Dinner

Spicy Spaghetti Squash Casserole

Fresh spinach, raw or cooked with ranch dressing drizzled on top

Day 28

- Breakfast

Full fat yogurt unsweetened with berries, chia seeds, flax seeds

- Lunch

Vegetarian chili with tomato, sour cream, a variety of beans and tomatoes

- Dinner

Zucchini spiral pasta noodles with creamy yogurt avocado sauce

Day 29

- Breakfast

Cauliflower "bread" grilled cheese sandwich (similar to cauliflower crust pizza but made as a grilled cheese sandwich instead.

- Lunch

Green beans with mushrooms and tomatoes with a chicken breast on the side

- Dinner

Grape tomato marinara on pasta noodles with parmigiano Reggiano cheese and fresh cracked pepper.

Day 30

- Breakfast

Egg taco shells filled with choice of vegetables

- Lunch

Baked crispy tofu steaks with a sesame seed crust on a bed of zucchini strips and spinach

- Dinner

Baked Spaghetti squash filled with roasted tomatoes and eggplant, topped with melted, crispy cheese

Chapter 7: What to Do Next

As you take all of this information forth with you, it may seem overwhelming to begin applying this to your own life. Remember, life is a process, and you do not need to expect perfection from yourself right away. By taking the first step-reading this book, you are already on your way to changing your life. If you fall off and find that you are back to your old ways, try to find inspiration in the pages of this book once again. If you find that you are unable to find success on your own, there is no shame in seeking professional help. There are many people who are trained professionals in dealing with disordered eating and who can serve as a mentor or a guide for you as you navigate this challenge.

How To Seek Help If It Becomes Uncontrollable?

Understanding and accepting that you need help is the first step to recovery. By reading this book, you have taken this step. If you need further help, there is no shame in accepting this fact. There are many ways to seek help for disordered eating, depending on the level of help that you need. Below is a list of ways that you can seek help, ordered from least to most help.

- Online resources
- Support System
- Support Group
- Group counseling
- Anonymous online counseling or telephone counseling
- One on One counseling

- Talk therapy
- Rehab centers

Counseling or Therapy

Talking therapies are very effective treatments for disordered eating. The things that people learn in therapy gives them the insight and skills in order to feel better and tackle their eating disorder, as well as to prevent it from coming back in the future.

One example of talk therapy is Cognitive Behavioral Therapy or CBT. The way that cognitive behavioral therapy works is by putting an emphasis on the relationship between a person's thoughts, emotions, and behaviors. The theory behind this is that when a person changes any one of these components, change will be initiated in the others. The goal of CBT is to help a person decrease negative thoughts or the amount of worry they experience in order to increase their overall quality of life.

If you think that this is something you would benefit from, please reach out to your local resources to find out more.

CPSIA information can be obtained
at www.ICGtesting.com
Printed in the USA
BVHW040935231220
596286BV00016B/66

9 781913 710965